# Persistent Fat Loss:

## Combining Ketosis and Intermittent Fasting for Year-Round Fitness

**Cristian Vlad Zot**

*Page left blank intentionally*

*Note to the reader (disclaimer)*

The information from this book is intended to describe the possible benefits of combining nutritional ketosis with intermittent fasting. However, if you decide to treat your illnesses, do it under the supervision of your physician. Do not use this book as a substitute for professional medical care or treatment.

Every effort has been made to ensure that the information contained in the book is complete and accurate. However, the author is not engaged in rendering advice to the individual reader.

This book should not serve as a how-to guide for therapeutic, periodic, and/or intermittent fasting. If you decide to follow such endeavors, do it under the supervision of a qualified physician.

# Table of Contents

Persistent Fat Loss

# Introduction

You know you're onto something when you see it's been working for you for so long! For me, I wouldn't say it's been that long. I've only been using the combination of nutritional ketosis and intermittent fasting to remain lean year round since January 2014. Hopefully, this strategy is not going to fail me any time soon.

If you don't know what ketosis or intermittent fasting is, don't worry. This is what this guide is for. But let me start by introducing myself.

It was the summer of 2013...

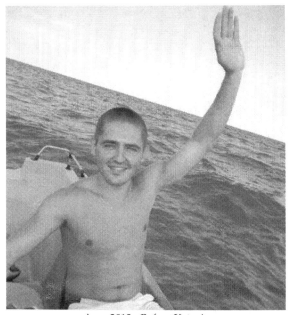

Aug. 2013 - Before Ketosis

At that time I was a fit person, but, to my satisfaction, my abdominal muscles were not visible enough. I've been trying for three years (since 2010) to lose the last few inches of fat from my abdominal area, but my efforts did not pay off.

I experimented with low-calorie diets, with increasing my protein intake, and with the Slow Carb Diet of Tim Ferriss. The stubborn fat would not come off.

I think that all diets or nutritional approaches can work, as long as you tailor them to your individual needs. But, when you're a perfectionist and you don't settle with the label 'fit' and you purpose for a visible 'six pack', you may have to take things to a superior level.

To give you a baseline, here's a different version of myself:

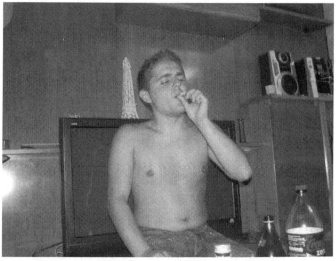

Summer of 2008

I wrote the details of fat loss journey in my first book Ketone Power. I will only give you a brief version here because the purpose of this book is to serve as a guide to help you adapt my strategy for your health optimization purposes.

To make a long story short, I started using nutritional ketosis in late September 2013. In a 2 month period I went from 19.6% bodyfat to ~14.4% bodyfat. I used a DEXA scanner to measure my body composition.

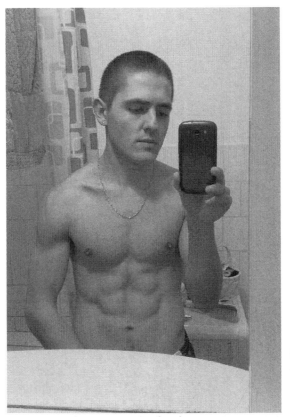

Dec. 2013 - 2 Months of Ketosis

In a few words, ketosis is the metabolic state where your body predominantly uses fats and ketones (fat derived metabolites) for energy, instead of sugar. This state is not easy to sustain.

Then, in early 2014 I started using the second strategy that you will learn about in this book, which is Intermittent Fasting (IF).

IF is a protocol that promotes food consumption during a feeding-window of 8 hours (or less) and uses a fasting window of at least 16 hours.

With IF you fast for 16 hours a day, and then you consume all your food in the remaining 8 hours. I personally fast for at least 18 hours everyday and consume food in the remaining 6 hours. Since 2014 I've been using these two strategies together and I've been able to maintain my body composition as you can see in the following images:

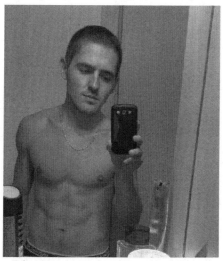

Feb. 2014 - 2 Months of IF and 5 of Ketosis

Persistent Fat Loss

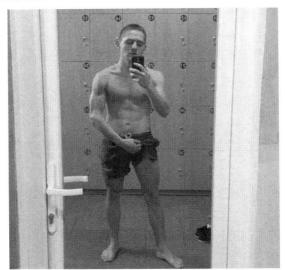

Oct. 2014 - 10 Months of IF and 13 of Ketosis

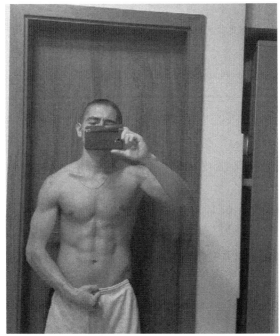

July 2015 - 19 Months of IF and 22 of Ketosis

Persistent Fat Loss

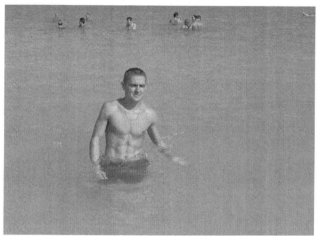

Oct. 2015 - 22 Months of IF and 25 of Ketosis

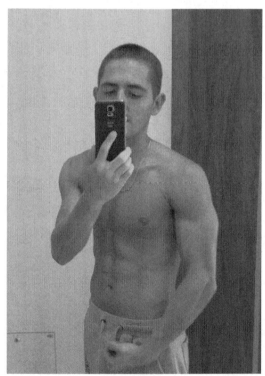

October 2015

Hopefully, these pictures caught your attention and proved the consistency that I got with the combination of ketosis and intermittent fasting. My purpose with this guide is for you to be able to adapt and implement these strategies and to obtain similar, if not better, results.

## What you get out of this book

You will learn about ketosis, ketogenic diets, and the process keto-adaptation. You will become familiar with the practice of intermittent fasting and with my 18/6 protocol. Throughout the book, I will use my journey as an example. And I will show you how to combine ketosis and intermittent fasting for enhanced fat loss. This is the major theme of the book.

Then I will provide some meal examples, and I will start with the ones that I use. You will be able to design your own meals as you learn the underlying principles.

I will teach you how to exercise with weights and your own bodyweight. Then you will learn about the tools that I'm using to track my journey and constantly improve my results.

Last but not least, I will provide further directions so that you can tailor this approach to your individual needs.

## The structure of the book and how you should read it

I have structured this book in chapters and lessons. As you progress through the lessons you will know the most important details and take away messages from the 2 strategies. Each lesson builds on top of the previous lessons. And many lessons are action oriented, so I would recommend that you implement the concepts as you go along.

This book is somewhat different from my first four books in which I quote science and research articles with every phrase. You do not need to have prior medical or technical knowledge to read this book because I purposed it to be written in lay terms.

I want to give you a small offer in case you want to digest the content of this guide in a book format, where you have colleagues and you can help each other in your fat loss endeavor. It is also the place where I can provide feedback to your journey. So, here is a 50% discount coupon for my book on ketosis and intermittent fasting:

http://bit.ly/persistcourse

Before starting with the first chapter, I would like you to read this important message:

*None of the content in this book should be taken as medical advice. It should not be used as a substitute for professional medical care or treatment. I am not a doctor and I don't play one on the Internet either; if you decide to implement any strategy, protocol, or therapy discussed or presented here, you do it on your own risk and you should do it under the supervision of a qualified physician/authority.*

# Chapter 1:
## Introduction to Ketosis and Intermittent Fasting

In the first chapter of the book I will introduce to you ketosis (nutritional ketosis) as a metabolic state and Intermittent Fasting as a strategy for timing your meals. Each of these methods alone is very powerful at shedding pounds, so you may imagine what a combination of the two can result in, provided that the overall strategy is well formulated.

Many people have been able to maximize fat loss in this way. I am one of them. And this is the major theme of the book.

This chapter discusses:

1. Different Metabolic States
2. The Metabolic State of Most People
3. Macronutrients 101 - And Food Examples
4. Ketosis as a Metabolic State
5. What Implies Ketosis
6. How to Measure Ketosis
7. Carbohydrate Intake for Ketosis
8. When Fasting Enters the Scene
9. Different Types of Intermittent Fasting (+My Approach)

So, let's get straight into the first lesson.

Persistent Fat Loss

## Lesson 1 - Different Metabolic States

Simplistically speaking, humans have two major built-in metabolic mechanisms. One is fueled by glucose, which is the end product of breaking down the carbohydrates that you eat and another one that is fueled by the fat you eat and the fat you have stored in your adipose tissue.

From a macronutrient perspective, food consists of three major groups: carbohydrates, proteins, and fats.

Carbohydrates are broken down into glucose and are used to fuel a sugar based metabolism. Some carbohydrates are indigestible and feed the gut microbes (bacteria inside your large intestines), while others are more complex and it takes more time to break them down into glucose.

Proteins are broken down into amino-acids and are used as building blocks inside the body.

Fats are broken down into fatty acids and glycerol. It is easier for you body to break down carbohydrates and use glucose for fuel. They are less energy-dense, as you will learn in an upcoming lesson.

When you do not consume sufficient carbohydrates to be in the glucose based metabolism efficiently or when you fast (when you do not eat for longer periods of time), your body will break down fatty acids from food or from you adipose tissue and make ketone bodies in the liver.

These ketone bodies (also known as ketones) serve as fuel for the brain and for many cells inside the body. There are three ketone bodies: beta-hydroxybutyrate, acetoacetate, and acetone. You do not need to memorize these medical terms.

In this fat-powered metabolism, your body runs predominantly on fatty acids and ketone bodies, and to a very little extent on glucose made inside the body, through a process called gluconeogenesis (endogenous glucose production).

In the next lesson you will learn about macronutrients and the way in which food is characterized by its macronutrient content. If you are new to nutrition, this lesson will be most helpful.

## Lesson 2 - Extra - Macros 101 - Food Examples

Food consists of macronutrients and micronutrients.

Macronutrients are: carbohydrates (or carbs), proteins, and fats. Micronutrients are: vitamins, minerals, phytochemicals, and many other trace nutrients.

The number of calories for each macronutrient: (this is important):

**1 g of protein = 4 kcals**
**1 g of carbohydrates = 4 kcals**
**1 g of fat = 9 kcals**

Fats are twice as rich in energy compared to the other two macronutrients (proteins and carbs). In this book I will use the terms *calories* (cal) and *kilocalories* (kcals) interchangeably.

Technology made it really easy to know the macronutrient and micronutrient content of each food. There are online applications such as *MyFitnessPal* and *Cronometer* (that we will use later in this guide) to tell you the caloric content, the macronutrient breakdown, the micronutrient content and other insightful information of any food out there.

In this book our main focus is on ketosis, ketogenic diets and intermittent fasting.

To reach/get into ketosis (the fat fueled metabolic state), you have to restrict the consumption of carbohydrates, moderate the consumption of proteins, and increase the consumption of fats. Please do not imagine that you will eat ridiculous amounts of bacon and butter. That is not reasonable.

For simplicity, I will provide a few examples of foods low and high in each of these macronutrients and in some combination of them.

**High carbohydrate**: bread, rice, some beans, potatoes, sweets, whole grain products, sweet fruits, sugar based products and the similar. These foods are low in fat as well.

**Low carb, high fiber, low fat**: vegetables, some beans, low-glycemic fruits (berries, lemons, grapefruit, etc).

**High fat, low carb**: cheese, bacon, coconut based foods, fatty meats, eggs (also high in protein), nuts (also high in protein), oils, butter, and similar products.

**High protein, low carb, low fat**: Lean meats, tofu, chick peas, protein powder, quinoa, cottage cheese, and many others.

Foods can exist in many other different combinations as well.

This was just an introductory list and should be used for reference purposes only. One can design a very well formulated diet for both sides of the spectrum (glucose based metabolism, fat based metabolism):

1. **A carbohydrate rich** diet that powers a glucose based metabolism.

2. A **very low carbohydrate diet** (ketogenic -> ketosis) that powers a fat based metabolism.

In this book we will focus on the latter.

More food types, macro partitioning examples and meal plans are to follow in later chapters of this book. In the next lesson you will learn about the metabolic state that most people use.

Persistent Fat Loss

## Lesson 2 - The Metabolic State of Most People

In the previous lesson I mentioned that there are two major metabolic states that you can be in:

- one in which the body is powered by glucose and
- one in which it uses ketones and fatty acids and it is powered by the fat from the diet and/or from the adipose tissue.

The later one is called ketosis or nutritional ketosis.

In ketosis, your brain uses ~70% ketones and the rest of energy is derived from glucose made inside the body. Conversely, when your body is powered by glucose, your brain uses 100% glucose.

In ketosis, the brain, the muscles, the heart and many cells in the body use ketones fatty acids predominantly. There are a few cell types that cannot use these metabolic substrates. They can only use glucose for energy and in ketosis that glucose is made inside the body through the process called gluconeogenesis (creation of new glucose).

Ketosis is not easy to achieve because one has to drastically restrict the consumption of carbohydrates. Some people need to consume less than 50g of carbohydrates per day to reach ketosis in a couple of days.

Others have to apply an even more restricted regime of less than 20g of carbohydrates per day (i.e. small slice of bread, 2.5 carrots, 2 medium size apples, or one big bowl of leafy green vegetables, etc.).

You can imagine why most people run predominantly on a glucose based metabolism. There's nothing wrong with that, as long as they consume a well formulated diet.

On another note ketosis can also be achieved by fasting (consuming nothing but water and non-caloric beverages). And this is one of the main interests of this book. In the next lesson I will tell you more about ketosis.

## Lesson 3 - Ketosis as Metabolic State

Ketosis, or nutritional ketosis, is the metabolic state where your body uses ketones and fatty acids for energy. I will repeat this for as long as it takes, because I want to make sure you are getting it right.

Ketosis can be achieved by drastically restricting the carbohydrates in your diet or by fasting.

To refresh your memory, most foods contain a different combination of the three macronutrients (carbs, fats, and protein), but in different ratios.

Some foods are higher in carbs and lower in fat (wheat based products, whole grain products, low-fat labeled products, etc.).

Others are higher in fat and lower in carbs (cheese, bacon, some nuts, oils, butter, and so on), while others are high in protein such lean cuts, protein powders, etc.

Combinations of foods containing all three macros are limitless.

Regardless of the diet you may follow, I would suggest avoiding foods that are both high in fats and high in carbs, such as processed foods, fast food, and the like. In this book, we will focus on consuming foods very low in carbohydrates, which are nutrient rich and energy rich.

To get into and to maintain the state of ketosis you have to consume ketogenic friendly foods, which are high in fat and low in carbs.

A few meal examples can combine a high-fat food with a low-carb food, such as:

- bacon with a plateful of leafy green vegetables, or
- eggs (high in fat high in protein) with a salad or with some vegetables (broccoli, kale, spinach, etc).

Later in this book I will show you how to design your meals more specifically.

Since ketosis is not easy to enter into and to maintain as a metabolic state, one has to be strict and has to quantify most of what they put in their mouths. Don't be scared though, it gets really easy after 2 or 3 weeks and after you learn the basics. Later on, ketosis can become a way of living. In the next short lesson, I will reiterate on the implications of ketosis.

## Lesson 4 - What Implies Ketosis

If you are not familiar with dieting, macronutrients, measuring food, and the like, it will be slightly challenging for the first two or three weeks on this protocol. That is the amount of time it takes to understand and to efficiently implement the basics.

If you are currently consuming a diet moderate or higher in carbohydrates (more than 50g per day), switching to ketosis means switching to a fat based metabolism, from a sugar (glucose) based metabolism.

You should understand that your body will need some time to adapt. When drastically reducing the carbohydrates in your diet, you will have to be consistent, that is: keep doing it everyday.

If you consume a diet very low in carbs today and tomorrow you eat many carbohydrate rich foods, you may never adapt to either of the two metabolisms. So you have to be strict.

But it all pays out. There are many advantages to ketosis if you are doing it right. I will talk about my own experience in future lessons.

**To get it straight, to enter into ketosis:**

1. Reduce carbohydrates to less than 50g per day.

2. Measure ketones (specifics, in the next lesson) to see if the initial restriction is enough.

If you are not in ketosis, restrict carbohydrate intake to less than 40g/day; measure ketones. Keep restricting until you reach ketosis. You can later readjust carbohydrate intake.

3. Once you reach ketosis, maintain the same dietary strategy and keep measuring ketones.

4. Spending more time in constant ketosis, improving the diet (optimizing for macronutrients and for micronutrients) will most likely lead to keto-adaptation and improved wellbeing.

Before moving on to the next lesson, I need to remind you that you will not be giving up your preferred foods if they are higher in carbohydrates.

Let's assume you love pizza; it is a carbohydrate rich food. Yet, it has many low-carbohydrate versions. It can be made to be ketogenic friendly.

In this way, it will not impact your ketosis status. Plus it may be healthier and better tasting. A low carbohydrate version of pizza would imply replacing the wheat based crust with a low-carbohydrate based crust made from almond flour, seed flour, nut flour, or any other low-carb flour.

Almost all carbohydrate rich foods have low-carb alternatives. So, you are not giving up anything when you decide to switch to long-term ketosis. That's one of the reasons I've been able to sustain this state for 2 years at the moment of this writing. For me, it's a lifestyle.

In the next lesson I will tell you how to measure ketosis.

## Lesson 5 - How to Measure Ketosis

There are several ways to measure ketosis. I will discuss the three most common. One of them measures urine ketones, another one measures blood ketones, while the third one measures breath ketones.

To measure urine ketones, you can use ketone sticks/strips - that's what they are called. Most of these sticks measure aceto-acetate, which is the ketone body used for energy creation inside the cell.

You can find these ketone sticks on Amazon for $10-$12 for 50 tests (search for "ketostix" and similar products). I have to mention that for some people urine sticks/strips may become less reliable after a while. As you get adapted to ketosis and your body becomes more efficient using ketones, you will excrete fewer of them in the urine.

For people like myself, they are still reliable even after 2 years of constant ketosis. I'm still dumping a lot of ketones in my urine.

One and probably the most reliable way to measure ketosis is through blood measurement devices. These blood monitors measure beta-hydroxybutyrate, which is the circulating form of ketones. They seem to be more reliable than urine measurements because they are not affected by the level of keto-adaptation. They are also more expensive, priced somewhere at $4-$5 per measurement.

To measure blood ketones you have to buy:

- the measuring device (on Amazon, search for "blood ketone monitor") and

- the strips for the device (on Amazon, search for "blood ketone strips").

Please make sure the strips are compatible with your blood ketone monitor. I personally did not use this type of measurement so far. I may use it in the future.

The third popular way to measure ketosis is by using a breath ketone meter (on Amazon, search for "breath ketone meter"). It should price somewhere at $100. It measures acetone, a ketone that is excreted from your body as you breathe out.

For a beginner, I'd recommend using the cheaper urine ketone strips.

Now that you know how to measure ketosis, you may be wondering about the absolute levels of ketones that define the state of ketosis.

I would say that whether you use urine or blood measurements, you are in ketosis when your levels are above 0.5 mmol/L.

An optimum range of ketosis would be between 2-5 mmol/L. For people who do not eat for longer periods of time (in situations like water only fasting) the level of ketones may go above this range, but it should not surpass 10-12 mmol/L.

Non-T1-diabetic persons (most normal people) may not worry about too many ketones in their body because they will also have some level of insulin secretion to keep the PH in a fairly good balance. We will discuss more about this in a future lesson on ketoacidosis.

One of the biggest mistakes people often make is that they do not go too low on carbohydrates so that they could start producing ketones. In this situation, they are still sugar burners, but very inefficient ones. Since your brain has very low sugar to derive energy from and since its not using ketones either, you will experience brain fog and low energy levels. That's why measuring ketones should be a must!

In the next lesson you will learn about the level of carbohydrate restriction that you have to go for in order to reach and to maintain ketosis.

Persistent Fat Loss

## Lesson 6 - Carbohydrate Intake for Ketosis

It is, mostly, carbohydrate restriction that is the determining factor for entering into and maintaining the state of ketosis. Protein restriction should also be considered, but it is not as important. I will discuss both.

For most people, consuming less than 50g of total carbohydrates is enough to enter ketosis in a few days and maintain it further. This happens gradually as the glycogen stored in the liver and in the muscles gets depleted.

I have to emphasize that even though fiber (which is a carbohydrate) is mostly indigestible, it is better to count it in for the total number (or amount) of carbohydrates you consume daily.

We are not interested in counting net carbohydrates (**total carbohydrates - fiber**), but total carbohydrates, which include fiber.

For some people who are more metabolically deranged or suffer from different diseases, they need to restrict carbohydrates even further, to less than 30g of total carbohydrates per day and in the worst cases to less than 20g of carbohydrates per day. These folks will mostly consume fatty foods and decent amounts of vegetables.

In this case, measuring ketosis is a must. You can use any of the methods that I discussed in our previous lesson.

Though not as important, protein intake should not be ignored. Consuming too much protein (more than 1.5g per kg of bodyweight) can have a negative impact on ketosis.

When too much protein is consumed and cannot be efficiently used for structural purposes, it will be inefficiently converted into glucose through the process of gluconeogenesis. And blood glucose levels are inversely correlated with ketone levels.

When BG is higher, ketones are lower: except for some cases (such as in people who suffer from T1 diabetes).

I, for example, weigh 142 pounds or ~66 kg. I usually consume between 50-80g of protein per day. This amount is below the threshold of 1.5g of protein per kg of bodyweight.

My gym performance is on a constant-improvement trend; so I believe some people do not have to consume increased amounts of protein to build and to maintain lean mass (that is, muscle).

Remember, each one of us is different. Hence, measuring ketosis should be a must. You have to find your own daily amount of carbs that you can consume to enter and to maintain this state.

I, for example, am fairly lean and I exercise regularly. I can consume up to 100g of total carbohydrates per day and still remain in ketosis (though I mostly consume less than 50g of total carbohydrates per day).

Conversely, other people need to go below 20g of total carbohydrates per day to stay in this state.

In the next lesson I will introduce you to the practice of intermittent fasting.

## Lesson 7 - When Fasting Enters the Scene

One of the great advantages for people who efficiently enter and stay in ketosis is its hunger suppression effect.

There are many positive aspects and potential advantages that ketosis allows for; and I will describe them in more detail in Chapter 2.

I was used to eating at least three times a day before doing ketosis back in late 2013. When I was 2-3 months in my practice of ketosis, in Dec. 2013, I was somewhat forcing myself to eat as often as I used to.

I was never hungry even when I was consuming fewer calories than my body *needed* everyday. That was when I started coping with the idea of fasting intermittently.

**Intermittent fasting** (IF) is the practice of restricting your meal intake to a window of a couple of hours everyday. With IF you fast for the major part of the day and then you consume all your calories during the feeding window.

As you may guess, intermittent fasting is composed of a fasting window and a feeding window.

In the fasting window you only consume water and non-caloric beverages (tea, black coffee, etc).

In the feeding window you (should try to) consume all your calories. You could have 1 ,2, 3 or even more meals during this window. It's up to you and to the way in which you design your strategy.

The most popular Intermittent Fasting protocol is, probably, the 16/8.

Persistent Fat Loss

- *16* stands for the amount of hours you fast (fasting window)
- *8* stands for the amount of hours in which you consume food.

IF in of itself brings additional advantages to ketosis, so you can imagine of the power of these two combined.

In the next lesson you will learn about the various types of Intermittent Fasting.

## Lesson 8 - Different types of Intermittent Fasting

I have mentioned earlier that the most popular IF strategy is the 16/8, where you fast (consume nothing but water and non-caloric beverages) for 16 hours and eat all your calories in the remaining 8 hours.

An example of the 16/8 protocol can be:

- **Eat** all your calories from 12 at noon until 8 P.M. (meal partitioning and the number of meals is up to you). This is the 8-hour feeding window
- **Fast** from 8 P.M. until 12 at noon the next day. This is the 16-hour fasting window.

This may be a very easy protocol to follow because you will be sleeping through the major part of your fast (which happens to be during the night).

Other people following the 16/8 protocol have their feeding window from 10 A.M. to 6 P.M. and then they fast from 6 P.M. until 10 A.M. the next day.

There are also other variations of IF protocols:

**14/12** - 14 hours of fasting, 12 hours of eating
**12/12** - 12 hours of fasting, 12 hours of eating - probably not so efficient
**18/6** - 18 hours of fasting, 6 hours of eating
**20/4** - 20 hours of fasting, 4 hours of eating - not easy
**22/2** - 22 hours of fasting, 2 hours of eating - even more difficult.

My personal approach is 18/6. However, there are many days when I fast for 20 to 22 hours and then consume my food during the remaining 2-4 hours, which is my feeding window.

As you can imagine, often times I cannot consume all my calories in such a short feeding window, so I remain in a caloric deficit, which is not a bad thing. It allows me to feast (over-consume calories) from time to time. I will provide more details on my personal strategy in Chapter 2.

Next stop, Chapter 2...

But first, please take a moment and try to see if you know the answer to the following questions. To verify your answers, you can find the key at the end of this book.

## Chapter 1 - Quiz

**1. What are the two major metabolic states that most people can be in?**

a) ketosis and keto-acidosis
b) ketosis and IF
c) ketosis and carbosis
d) glucose powered metabolism and fat powered metabolism

**2. How many kcals (calories) are in a gram of fat?**

a) 4 kcals
b) 5 kcals
c) 9 kcals
d) 3 kcals

**3. How many kcals (calories) are in a gram of protein?**

a) 4 kcals
b) 5 kcals
c) 9 kcals
d) 3 kcals

**4. What is ketosis?**

a) a metabolic state where fat becomes the major metabolic substrate
b) a metabolic state where carbohydrates become the major metabolic substrate
c) a metabolic state where protein becomes the major metabolic substrate
d) a pathologic state

**5. How many grams of carbohydrates should you consume per day as a starting point of ketosis?**

a) less than 200g
b) less than 150g
c) less than 100g
d) less than 50g

6. **What is the cheapest way to measure ketosis?**

a) with a blood meter
b) with a breath meter
c) with a urine test
d) with a stool test

7. **What is currently the most reliable way to measure ketones?**

a) with a breath meter
b) with a blood meter
c) with a urine test
d) with a stool test

8. **What is intermittent fasting (IF)?**

a) a strategy of exercise
b) a protocol for reducing carbohydrates in the diet
c) a protocol for reducing fats in the diet
d) a strategy for meal timing, containing a feeding window and a fasting window.

9. **What is the intermittent fasting protocol promoted in this book?**

a) IF of 16/8 with 16 hours of fasting and 8 hours of feeding
b) IF of 18/6 with 18 hours of fasting and 6 hours of feeding
c) IF of 20/4 with 20 hours of fasting and 4 hours of feeding
d) IF of 14/10 with 14 hours of fasting and 10 hours of feeding

## 10. What is the major theme of this book?

a) combining ketosis and intermittent fasting.
b) reducing the consumption of carbohydrate rich foods.
c) reducing the consumption of fats.
d) learning about prolonged fasting.

Persistent Fat Loss

# Chapter 2:
## Physiologic Aspects of Ketosis and IF
## A call for Personalized Approaches

Now that you're fairly familiar with ketosis as a metabolic state and with intermittent fasting as a strategy to time your meals, I want to go a bit further into the science of both of these strategies.

I will not stress you too much with technical terms though. Nevertheless, I want you to better understand the implications of these two protocols so that you can efficiently include them into your lifestyle.

In this chapter you will learn about:

1. Fat Intake and Ketosis
2. Common Mistakes People Make on Ketogenic Diets
3. Ketosis and Keto-Acidosis
4. Advantages of Ketosis
5. Disadvantages of Ketosis
6. The Process of Keto-Adaptation
7. My personal IF Protocol
8. IF and physiologic Adaptations
9. Long Term Intermittent Fasting
10. Combining IF and Ketosis

So, let's jump straight into the first lesson.

Persistent Fat Loss

## Lesson 1 - Fat Intake and Ketosis

I want to discuss about one of the biggest misconceptions that people have regarding long-term ketosis. I want you to get the best out of ketosis so I want to set this matter straight.

You have to avoid the common mistakes that many keto followers make. One of them involves the amount of fat you need or don't need to eat to maintain ketosis.

In Chapter 1 you learned that ketosis (nutritional ketosis) can be achieved by following a very-low-carbohydrate-moderate-protein diet or by fasting. As you can observe, fat intake was not mentioned in the sentence.

Fat is a very important macronutrient. It makes up for 60% of your brain's dry weight. It is found in the structure of almost all cell walls inside your body. It can have anti-inflammatory properties. There are a lot of advantages attached to it. Fat is also the substrate for ketones which are made in the liver through the process of ketogenesis.

But this does not mean that you have to eat ridiculous amounts of fat to be in ketosis. Many followers of the ketogenic diet seem to think so, which is why they may never achieved the optimal health they've been dreaming of.

Your body can use its own fat stores to power ketosis, provided that your carbohydrate and protein intake allow for that. Please keep this in mind.

From a personal perspective, I started as most people do. In the first few months of ketosis I probably consumed ~80% of my calories from fat.

Persistent Fat Loss

At that time I was eating ~2,500kcals/day:

80% of 2,500 = 2,000 kcals from fat alone.
1g of fat is 9 kcals => I was consuming ~220g of fat per day.

That seems a lot now. Later, I optimized my diet by consuming more vegetables and plant foods, reducing calories (because I didn't feel like eating as many calories), and by reducing fat intake.

From a macronutrient perspective, I've been most consistent with consuming 60-65% of my calories coming from fat, while the rest of 18-23% from protein and the remaining 10-15% from carbohydrates. This is not set in stone though. I almost always change/tweak something.

Since I mostly consume between 1,500-1,700 kcals per day, 65% coming from fat is not as much. And since my diet is low-calorie (I reduced calories as I am never hungry - one of the potential benefits of ketosis), I can use both fats from my diet and from my own body stores to power ketosis.

The major take away that I want you to have from this lesson is that you do not have to go crazy about fat consumption to power ketosis. Reducing carbohydrates and moderating protein intake are more important, if you ask me.

In the next lesson I will briefly discuss other mistakes often made by people who use ketogenic diets.

# Lesson 2 - Common Mistakes People Make on Ketogenic Diets

To reiterate, one of the biggest mistakes made by many folks following a ketogenic diet is that they consume too much fat.

**Another common mistake** that I often see is that they go onto these so-called *'fat fasts'*.

You now know what fasting is all about - consuming nothing but water and non-caloric beverages.

A *'fat fast'* is a strategy to consume nothing but 1,000 kcals of fat everyday for a couple of days, hoping this will kick-boost ketosis. The major requirement for ketosis involves reducing carbohydrate intake and moderating protein intake. Hence, the concept of fat fasting may be regarded as absurd.

It provides no additional benefit to *water-only* fasting. Eating pure fat has no magic attached to it, even though some folks would like to think so. However, this strategy may be helpful for people who want to get into ketosis really quick and do not feel comfortable doing *water-only fasting* for multiple days in a row. From a personal standpoint, I would not use *fat-fasting*.

Instead, I would reduce carbohydrates, progressively increase fat intake up to a certain level, and progressively decrease caloric intake as hunger comes down naturally as you start adapting to ketosis.

For people coming from a high-carbohydrate diet it may take a few days to get into ketosis because they have to deplete their body glucose stores (glycogen). What I suggested above may seem more rational than fat-fasting.

**Another common mistake** is the belief that you can consume as many calories as you want on a ketogenic diet because since you are in ketosis, you will not get fat.

While it may be somewhat true that consuming more calories in ketosis leads to an increased metabolic rate, it may be challenging (if I may) to think that over-consuming calories over the long-term will not lead to weight gain, regardless of the nutritional protocol and the metabolic state you are in.

**Too much protein** consumption is another trap that folks fall into. For structural purposes, your body may do with as little as 0.8g of protein per KG of bodyweight, while some studies show efficient muscle building with as little as 1g of protein per KG (not pound) of bodyweight.

Purposing for 1-1.5g of protein per KG of bodyweight would be rational if you want to build more lean mass.

**Another mistake** is that people going on a ketogenic diet consume too much fat and very few carbohydrates. From my perspective it is important to consume greens, vegetables and plant foods in decent amounts. Most folks will not get kicked out of ketosis from the carbohydrates in these plant foods. Grains, rice, and potatoes should be avoided all together, though.

**Another irrational strategy** for people following ketogenic diets is to put oils and butter in their coffee in the thought they will boost their ketosis or improve their mental state. From my perspective this is one way to increase the energy content of your diet (increase calories) without optimizing for nutrient intake - too much fat, too few nutrients.

**Another mistake involves** alcohol intake. I will dedicate a separate lesson for this topic.

Avoiding these common mistakes may put you on a faster pace to improving your wellbeing with ketosis and IF. In the next lesson you will learn about the difference between ketosis and keto-acidosis.

Persistent Fat Loss

## Lesson 3 - Ketosis and Keto-Acidosis

Ketosis got a bad fame in the medical and in the nutritional community due to a pathologic (and not metabolic) state with a similar name but a different context - that is keto-acidosis.

**Ketosis**, also known as **nutritional ketosis**, is the metabolic state where your body uses ketones and fatty acids to create energy. Blood ketone levels in nutritional ketosis fall between 0.5 and 10 mmol/L.

Mild ketosis starts at 0.5 mmol/L while the optimal ketone zone may fall between 2-5 mmol/L. Some experts in the community like to call this - the sweet spot.

Fasting for several days - that is consuming nothing but water - raises ketone levels to ~10 mmol/L. Your body still produces insulin in minute amounts.

Conversely, **ketoacidosis** is the pathologic state where your blood ketone levels reach 20 mmol/L or more, while insulin production does not occur to counterbalance this acidic state.

This is usually the case for Type 1 Diabetes, when people with this condition produce too many ketones and cannot produce insulin to regulate/balance this process. They require insulin administration to live a decent life.

For most healthy people, ketoacidosis does not occur, even if you fast for 40 days or more. If you use nutritional ketosis and if you design your diet optimally (to include both healthy fats and decent amounts of vegetables and plant foods along with moderate protein consumption), you will have no issue with keto-acidosis or its possible negative consequences.

Persistent Fat Loss

In the next lesson you will learn about the possible benefits of ketosis.

## Lesson 4 - Advantages of Ketosis

If done correctly, ketosis can provide many benefits.

One of the advantages that most people report (and that I have personally experienced) is **hunger suppression.**

When your body learns that it can rely on fat drawn from its own adipose tissue and does not have to worry about the fast metabolizing and the short storage of glucose within the body, and most importantly, when your brain learns to efficiently use ketones, hunger tends to fade away. The panic mode (eating every 3-4 hours) is gone. The change in the signaling of different hormones allows for this adaptation.

**Another advantage** attached to ketosis is higher energy levels. I have felt like this from the very second week of ketosis. Uninterrupted flow of energy day-in day-out.

However, you do have to consider the initial adaptation period of days to weeks, when your energy levels may be extremely low and you may experience brain fog. After all, your body switches to a different metabolic substrate. Most folks quit ketosis as they don't want to push through this initial uncomfortable adaptation period.

**A third advantage** may refer to cognitive improvement: not feeling the mid-day after-lunch mental and energy crash; having constantly higher brain performance the entire day.

**Another advantage** that many people report is quicker recovery after workouts, as well as higher exercising performance, especially for endurance athletes. Burning fat may be more advantageous and less demanding in strenuous endurance competitions.

Most of us carry at least 30,000 - 40,000 kcals stored in our adipose tissue. For reference, a marathon's energy requirements are around 3,000 - 4,000 kcals. Your body's glucose stores (glycogen) are ~1,600 - 2,000 kcals, meaning that if you use glucose as your primary fuel you will have to consume glucose rich foods and beverages during your competition. Otherwise, you will run out of energy.

If you run on fat and your fat store is at least 30,000 kcals (for lean individuals), you will require nothing but water and some electrolytes to get the competition to an end.

High-intensity training and strength training can also derive advantages from ketosis. But they require adapting to a ketosis protocol (ketogenic diet) for the long term. My personal strategy is an example of that. I will discuss about this in further details in a future lesson.

There are many more advantages to ketosis. Some of them will be mentioned throughout this book while the rest, well... I will let you discover them for yourself.

In the next lesson I will discuss some of the possible disadvantages of ketosis.

## Lesson 5 - Disadvantages of Ketosis

**Most of the disadvantages** of ketosis may appear due to an inappropriate approach to adopting this protocol; and also due to some possible genetic mutations that may prevent the body from efficiently entering into and maintaining this state.

First of all, people who consumed a high-carbohydrate diet all their life may find it challenging to enter into ketosis. You can imagine that it is not easy to instantly switch to a different metabolic substrate - to a fat based metabolism from a carbohydrate based metabolism.

Signs and symptoms of glucose withdrawal might appear in this case. Some examples are: brain fog, light headedness, cold limbs, low energy levels, sugar cravings, increased hunger, and a few others.

One would have to push through these symptoms to enter into and to maintain ketosis. These symptoms are temporary and may go away after a few days. Consuming sufficient water and electrolytes and eating nutrient rich foods may help during the process.

Switching to ketosis from a glucose based metabolism involves the creation of different enzymes to power the fat based metabolism. It also involves the creation of more mitochondria (which are the powerhouses of your cells), and the adaptation of your brain to using predominantly ketones, instead of glucose.

**Another possible disadvantage** to ketosis, for some people, is the inflexible amount of carbohydrates they can consume. If they are used to eating many carbohydrate rich foods, this may be an impediment.

But you have to remember that I mentioned that for every high-carbohydrate food there is at least 1 very-low-carb (keto-friendly) alternative.

**Another possible disadvantage** is that ketosis needs to be maintained over the long-term for efficiency in high-intensity and strength-training; and also for many other of its benefits.

And for many folks this is another impediment. But, as with any strategy, I'd recommend consider this as a lifestyle approach (like I did) and not just as a temporary strategy.

There may be some other possible disadvantages to ketosis; but in my opinion, these are the most important to be addressed. In the next lesson I will talk about the process of keto-adaptation.

## Lesson 6 - The Process of Keto-Adaptation

Keto adaptation is the process by which you adhere/adapt to ketosis (nutritional ketosis) over the long-term.

Short-term keto-adaptation can take anywhere between 2 to 4 weeks of constant ketosis. It provides some of the benefits of ketosis that I mentioned earlier.

Short-term ketosis (cyclically) has been used with great success by many people. For example, bodybuilders use it when "cutting". As they want to lose fat and get shredded for competition, they go on a ketogenic diet for a couple of weeks.

Long-term keto-adaptation is more tedious and it may involve more than 6-12 or even 18 months of ketosis. This is when one will adapt to efficiently burn fatty acids and ketones for energy and this is also when all the benefits of ketosis may be experienced.

You can imagine that since you will be going in this state for a long time, you have to design a well formulated diet in which you optimize not only for macronutrients, but also for micronutrient intake.

In long-term ketosis it would not be rational or optimal to consume ridiculous amounts of fat, like many *weekend keto warriors* tend to mistakenly do.

It would be more rational to consume decent amounts of healthy fats, decent amounts of vegetables and plant foods, and moderate amounts of protein. Once again, I call for rationality and not for insanity. I want you to take this strategy as responsibly as possible.

Coming from a high-carb-diet background, it would require you to go through a few critical days and the symptoms that I mentioned earlier to enter into ketosis. Once you reach ketosis, it would be advised to maintain it over the long-term.

If for some reason you consume a high-carbohydrate food that kicks you out of ketosis or if you consume too much alcohol, please do not stress yourself with this. Learn from your mistakes and start-over.

A day out of ketosis should not be a problem if you stayed in ketosis for long enough for your body to adapt to this metabolic state.

All of us have bad days, days in which we fall off the wagon. We have to take them with a grain of salt, and move on without blaming us for what happened. Learning from mistakes is the key. And it's even better when you can learn from the mistakes of other people.

For personal reference, I've been in constant ketosis for more than 2 years (since the fall of 2013). I've been kicked out of ketosis a couple of times. It did not impact my long-term strategy.

It took a couple of months of constant ketosis to recover my performance in the gym (lifting weights) and in my kickboxing practice. I refer to the performance I had when I consumed a higher carbohydrate diet.

That's why to be fully optimal in ketosis, long-term keto-adaptation may represent the approach that you should target for.

In the next lesson you will learn about my personal intermittent fasting strategy.

## Lesson 7 - My Personal IF Protocol

Previously, you learned that the most popular intermittent fasting strategy is the 16/8, that is fasting for 16 hours and eating during the remaining 8-hour feeding window.

My strategy is a bit more advanced and it is also the strategy that I propose to you, but not necessarily from the very beginning.

My IF protocol is 18/6, that is 18 hours of fasting and 6 hours of eating. I follow this protocol almost everyday. However, there are many variations and exceptions.

Sometimes I do 20/4 - 20 hours of fasting and 4 hours of eating and some other times I fast for 24 hours or even more. But for my 18/6 IF protocol, I consume food between 10 A.M. to 4 P.M. and then fast from 4 P.M. until the next day at 10 A.M.

This is convenient for me because when I'm at home (I travel quite often lately), I go to the gym at 7 A.M. When I return, I cook a big breakfast (I will talk about its content in a future lesson) which I consume at 10 A.M. Then I have a big snack at 3 P.M. which lasts for about an hour, until 4 P.M.

So, I basically have 2 meals per day most of the days. When I fast for 24 hours or more, I only have 1 very large meal. There are some days when I do not fast the 18/6 way and I consume more than 2 meals. But these days are exceptional/situational days.

If you have never engaged in IF, I'd recommend starting with a 14/10 IF protocol, where you fast for 14 hours, and consume food in the remaining 10 hours. An example could be eating from 10 A.M. to 8 P.M. and then fasting from 8 P.M. until the next day at 10 A.M. This should not be difficult, and during the feeding window you could keep your 3 meal/day protocol if that's the one you're currently following.

As you get used to it, you can progress into the more efficient IF protocols. The next logical step would be to do the 16/8 with 3 meals during the feeding window, followed by the 16/8 with 2 meals.

Then you could progress into 18/6 with 2 meals and see how you handle it. And then you could experiment from time to time with 20/4 with 2 meals, 22/2 with 1 meal, or even 24 hours fasting with 1 meal post-fast.

Keep in mind that no matter the IF strategy you follow, you should always try to consume all your calories for the day. Most of the time you will be so satisfied that you will not be able to do eat to your daily required caloric intake. This is convenient if you're on a fat loss track. And it also leaves a lot of room for planned feasting days. But, more on this later.

In the next lesson, I will discuss about the physiologic adaptations that occur under the more advanced IF protocols, such as the 16/8, 18/6, 20/4, and 24.

## Lesson 8 - IF and Physiologic Adaptations

When you start practicing intermittent fasting and you do it consistently, there are several metabolic and hormonal adaptations that take place inside your body. Without burdening you too much with biochemistry and medical terminology, I will try to explain in lay terms how some of your hormones change their signaling behavior and how this may have an impact on your wellbeing.

When you do IF with a fasting window of at least 16 hours:

- several hours into your fasting window insulin secretion goes down
- lower insulin levels will allow for fatty acids to be released from the adipose tissue and be used for energy
- lower insulin levels will also reduce hunger
- growth hormone secretion can increase 2,000%, further promoting fatty acid metabolism and lean mass preservation, as well as muscle build-up (given that you exercise appropriately)
- IGF-1, a signaling factor characteristically higher in cancer, is reduced drastically
- mTOR, another growth factor characteristic of cell proliferation is also reduced significantly

Ghrelin is a hunger hormone released near meal time which increases your appetite and prepares your body for taking in food. Its secretion goes down after you eat. If you practice IF and have a fairly regular feeding window, you may only get hungry around meal time.

For example, if my feeding window of 6 hours is between 10 A.M. and 4 P.M. and I consume 2 meals, one at 10 A.M. and the second one at 3 P.M., ghrelin will be secreted around those hours to increase my appetite and prepare my body for food intake. I will not have appetite surges or hunger pangs outside this timeframe. To be more specific, with my protocol I am never hungry at night because I got my body to get used to this meal timing regime.

There are also many other important hormones and regulating factors (leptin, CCK, POMC, etc) that change with IF, but for the sake of keeping this lesson straight and to the point, I only mentioned the ones from above.

In the next lesson you will learn about long-term intermittent fasting.

## Lesson 9 - Long Term Intermittent Fasting

Same as with ketosis, I would advise you to adopt IF as a long-term strategy. Not only that it elicits many more benefits than it would if you do it sort-term, but it is also easier to adhere to it and to make it part of a better lifestyle.

One of the possible advantages is the control over your feeding and fasting behavior. With IF you know that you're only going to eat during your feeding window (whatever that is).

This will minimize for unplanned intake of food, and inefficient snacking all throughout the day. You will have better control over the amount of food you consume and you could easily plan your day according to your meal timing protocol.

Of course, from time to time you can allow for exceptions, such as having dinner with a friend - dinner that is not in your feeding window, if your feeding window occurs during the first part of the day. But these exceptions are what they are, exceptions and not the rule.

Long-term intermittent fasting will allow for increased satisfaction when you consume food, especially if you fast for 20 hours and then try to consume all your calories within a 4 hour window.

Most of the time you will not be able to do that because you will reach satiety before reaching your required daily caloric intake.

Another possible advantage is that as you adapt to the protocol, you will burn more fat every day - as you progress a couple of hours into your fasting window. If you consume food every 3-4 hours, you may never be able to efficiently tap into your body fat stores. The constantly high insulin secretion will keep you hungry.

Long-term IF can also be seen as a disadvantage because you will not be able to eat whenever you want. You will only consume food during your feeding window, with the few exceptions that I discussed above. So, it depends on how you view it.

Personally, I've been doing intermittent fasting since January 2014 almost every day (more than 95% of the time). I've never been more satisfied and adherent to the way I eat. I achieved my physiologic goals ever since the very beginning so I've been in maintenance mode almost all this time. I consume comfort foods everyday (dark chocolate, cheese, and nuts) and I will discuss this in more detail in a future lesson.

In the next lesson I will tell you about the *'killer'* combination of ketosis and intermittent fasting.

## Lesson 10 - Combining IF and Ketosis

We are quite advanced into this book and so far you have become fairly intimate with the specifics of both of these two practices: ketosis and intermittent fasting. So, let's keep on rolling!

### What happens when you combine them? How to start?

First of all, I'd recommend you may start by implementing ketosis alone. It is going to be easier if you come from a moderate to low carbohydrate nutrition background, while it may be a bit more challenging if in the past you've been following a higher-carbohydrate diet. However, even if it's more challenging, it's not impossible to adopt ketosis in either of the situations.

To enter into ketosis, you may gradually reduce carbohydrates (for a couple of days) until you reach 50g of total carbohydrates per day. I recommend saving your carbohydrates for vegetables and plant foods. 50g of total carbohydrates per day allows for a decent amount of these foods.

Then I will recommend gradually increasing your fat intake to 70% of your calories.

For example, if you're a male and you desire to consume 2,000 kcals/day (many men will lose weight at this caloric intake), you will be consuming 70% of 2,000 = 1,400 kcals from fat alone. I'd recommend that for your fat intake you consume healthy fats from eggs, organs meats, fatty fish, coconut based foods, nuts, and a few others.

I also recommend moderating your protein intake to no more than 1.5g of protein per kg of bodyweight (that is ~0.8g of protein per pound bodyweight).

Once you maintain this strategy for a few days, start measuring ketosis with one of the methods mentioned in Lesson 5 of Chapter 1 (urine, blood, or breath). I'd recommend the urine strips since they are cheaper and work well for people starting with ketosis.

If you reach ketosis with this strategy, keep it going and don't change anything. Keep measuring ketones from time to time just to make sure you are maintaining it. If you are not in ketosis, you may further reduce carbohydrates to 40g per day, and then to 30g per day until you start measuring good levels of ketones in your body.

Once you've achieved ketosis, you should keep your strategy until you become fairly comfortable with it. After a couple of weeks, you will most likely start seeing the benefits that I mentioned in previous lessons, one of which is the aggressive hunger suppression effect of ketones.

When you reach this level, you can start implementing an IF protocol. As I recommended earlier, 14/10 with 3 meals during your feeding window should be easy to implement.

Once that becomes easy enough, you can progress to an IF of 16/8 with 3 meals, and further to an IF of 16/8 with 2 meals. When this becomes easy, you may adopt the protocol that I'm currently using, that is IF of 18/6 with 2 meals.

In a future lesson, I will be more specific about the foods that I use with this IF protocol and how you can adopt and adapt my strategy to your personal lifestyle.

Before moving on to Chapter 3, let's get you into a quick knowledge review...

## Chapter 2 - Quiz

### What is one of the biggest misconceptions of ketosis?

a) fat consumption has to be drastically increased
b) eating is only permitted after 4 P.M.
c) eating is only permitted before 6 P.M.
d) fat consumption has to be drastically reduced

### What is one of the major requirements for entering and maintaining ketosis?

a) drastically reducing protein intake
b) drastically reducing fat intake
c) drastically reducing protein and fat
d) drastically reducing carbohydrate intake.

### What is one of the major mistakes people do when on a ketogenic diet?

a) the belief that you can consume as many calories as you want
b) the belief that you have to eat more than 2g of protein per kg of bodyweight per day
c) the belief that protein intake should be very low
d) the belief that carbohydrates are evil

### What is one of the advantages of ketosis?

a) decreased libido
b) decreased appetite and hunger
c) that you can consume as much food as you want
d) that you will start feeling great from the very first day of this lifestyle

### What is one of the disadvantages of ketosis?

a) the possible longer period of time to efficiently adapt to this state
b) decreased appetite and hunger
c) decreased libido
d) that you cannot eat whatever you want

## What is the number of meals promoted for the IF strategy that you learn in this book?

a) 3 meals a day
b) 4 meals a day
c) 2 meals a day
d) 1 meal a day

## What is one of the requirements of any IF protocol?

a) to try to consume all your daily caloric requirements in your feeding window
b) to have at least 3 meals a day
c) to eat only in the evening
d) to stop alcohol consumption

## What is one of the misconceptions of IF?

a) that you have to stop alcohol consumption
b) that you have to follow a low calorie diet
c) that you have to consume a high-calorie diet
d) that you have to eat only 3 times per day

## What may be a good strategy for alcohol intake when combining ketosis and IF?

a) having alcohol during meal time
b) having alcohol prior to eating
c) having alcohol a couple of hours after eating
d) not having alcohol at all

**What is one of the physiologic adaptations that happens when doing IF for the long term?**

a) better insulin secretion
b) higher blood glucose levels
c) lower libido
d) lower growth hormone levels

Persistent Fat Loss

# Chapter 3:
## Getting Started - Concepts of Meal Prep and IF Protocols
## What to consume when Fasting

Now that you know much more about the concepts of IF and ketosis than most people, I will provide some more suggestions on how you can apply this knowledge and implement these two strategies in your own lifestyle. Additionally, you should be able to help others use these strategies to improve their own physiologies.

As a caveat, I need to mention that the reference strategy I will provide can and should be modified according to your own needs and preferences. You do not have to rigidly stick to the meal examples I provide here, nor with the exercising protocols that I talk about, or with my IF strategy. Personalizing your approach is a determining factor for long-term adherence.

In this chapter you will learn about:

1. The Most Used Foods to Enter and to Sustain Ketosis
2. My Personal Favorite Keto-Friendly Foods
3. How many Calories to Consume - How Many I consume
4. IF - Feeding Window - Earlier or Late in the Day
5. Getting Kicked of Ketosis for Too Much Food During IF's Feeding Window
6. Social Exceptions for IF
7. Fasting and Feasting - The Low-Calorie Advantage
8. Alcohol Intake - And my Personal Strategy

Now, let's start with the first lesson where I will be discussing the most common foods people consume to maintain ketosis.

Persistent Fat Loss

## Lesson 1 - The Most Used Foods to Enter and to Sustain Ketosis (+my personal favorites)

The popular approach to enter into ketosis is to start consuming significant amounts of fatty foods and drastically reducing carbohydrates. In my approach and in what you're about to learn, I want to leave room for more common sense.

The second layer of the nutritional approach to ketosis is to try to minimize food allergies, in case you have them.

**Some keto friendly foods high in fat (some of them high in protein) are:**

- whole eggs*, nuts*, seeds, fatty meat, fatty fish, fish oil, coconut based foods (coconut milk, coconut oil, coconut flakes, coconut flour), nut flours*, lard, beef tallow, olive oil, olives, peanuts*, peanut butter*, non-processed meat products, full fat Greek yoghurt, cheese, cottage cheese, aged cheese and most other cheeses, full fat milk*, almond milk, butter, ghee, sour cream, heavy cream, cream cheese, mozzarella, etc.

**Some keto friendly foods, very low in carbohydrates, are:**

- most green vegetables and plant foods - broccoli, kale, cauliflower, asparagus, green beans, some lentils, onion, green bell peppers, tomatoes*, mushrooms, Brussels sprouts, celeriac, pumpkin, turnips, artichoke, squash, spinach, lettuce, parsley root, radishes, cabbage, sauerkraut, pickles, chard, garlic, eggplant, zucchini, cucumbers, avocado, berries, lemons, grapefruits, limes, very dark chocolate, etc.

**Some keto friendly beverages are:**

- water obviously, coffee and tea (unsweetened or sweetened with stevia), red dry wine, spirits (hard alcoholic beverages), etc. Please avoid highly processed and sugar/syrup sweeten beverages.

**Foods that you should avoid completely:**

- all highly processed foods (with more than 2-3 ingredients on the ingredient list), all grain based and grain derived products, sweets, low-fat labeled foods (they are usually sugar added), beer, cocktails, sugary alcoholic drinks, soda, soda pop, high-glycemic fruits (sweet fruits), soy products, etc.

The foods marked with * are potentially allergenic, so I'd recommend avoiding them at first, at least until you get on track with your strategy. Subsequently, you can experiment with each of them, one at a time, and see how your body reacts.

Besides the foods I mentioned, there are many other foods that you can use to sustain ketosis. The only requirement is for them to fit within your carbohydrate limit for the day.

I recommend avoiding most foods coming with labels. But if you purchase a processed product, please make sure it does not contain additives, unnatural coloring agents, preservatives, and added sugar.

For example, I buy hard salami. But it only contains 5 ingredients: ground meat, salt, pepper, natural condiments, and natural membrane. Nothing unnatural here.

It is very easy to find and determine the macronutrient - and micronutrient - content for all the foods I listed here. There are many programs, websites and apps that you can install on your phone to help you with that. Two examples are *MyFitnessPal* and *Cronometer*.

I will show you how to use Cronometer in a future lesson. It is free and you can determine your starting and maintenance strategy for ketosis. It is an easy way to stay within your carbohydrate and caloric daily limits.

I highly suggest that you include decent amounts of vegetables and plant foods in your diet everyday because they add to the amount of micronutrients and phytochemicals that help you optimize your wellbeing.

Please do not obsess about fat consumption. It is important to consume healthy fats everyday. But consuming should not mean abusing.

I also suggest focusing not only on reducing carbohydrates, but also on moderating protein intake. This is another call for common sense.

In the next lesson I will tell you about my personal favorite ketogenic friendly foods.

Persistent Fat Loss

## Lesson 2 - My Personal Favorite Keto-Friendly Foods

In this lesson I will give you an overview of how I plan and what I eat during any particular day. This is not what I eat everyday though, so you should only take it as a situational example.

I usually workout in the morning, early - around 7 A.M. I lift heavy for ~an hour.

**I have a big breakfast at ~10 A.M. It contains:**

- 3 whole eggs
- 2 oz. bacon
- 1 tsp lard

I cook the eggs and bacon in lard.

- 5 oz coleslaw
- 2 oz tomato
- 1 tsp vinegar
- 1 tsp olive oil
- salt
- pepper

The vinegar, olive oil, salt and pepper are used as salad dressing.

- 2 oz. of red beans sprinkled with salt and pepper. Some people should avoid beans whenever starting a ketogenic diet as they may be kicked out of ketosis. You can experiment with consuming them later on.

**At 3 P.M. I have a big snack containing:**

- 1.6 oz 85% dark chocolate
- 3 oz. mixed nuts and seeds (almonds, cashews, walnuts, Brazil nuts, sunflower seeds, and peanuts*).
- 1 oz. hard cheese
- 4 oz. full fat Greek yoghurt.

People with nut and peanut allergies should avoid consuming them altogether.

I drink purified water, tomato juice* (unsweetened), lemon juice, grapefruit juice, and stevia sweetened coffee with ~1 oz. of whole milk.

With this example strategy, I am below 50g of total carbohydrates per day. I could consume up to 100g of total carbs per day because I will most likely not be kicked out of ketosis. But this is the strategy I got myself used to. I may change it in the future.

In Chapter 3 we will have a lesson where I plug these foods into *Cronometer* (the food tracking app we will be using) so that you can have an idea about it and be able to start using it yourself.

In the next lesson I will discuss about **daily caloric intake**.

## Lesson 3 - How Many Calories to Consume - How Many I Consume

If you do not know how many calories you are currently consuming everyday, here you will learn how to find that out.

Once you know how much you eat in any particular day, I'd recommend using that same number of calories for ketosis and the ketogenic diet you are switching to.

You can later reduce/adjust calories if you feel over-satisfied or if you feel that you are eating too much.

It would be unwise to give you a specific number of calories that you should consume everyday because we are all different and we all have different energy requirements everyday. Additionally to that, the hormonal behavior of each of us calls for different metabolic and energetic demands.

The only, somewhat accurate, way to find out how many calories you need in a specific day would be to spend 24 hours in a metabolic chamber (which is very uncomfortable and mostly unavailable - at the moment - for the wide public).

Daily total caloric suggestions for normal adult males, with moderate activity, fall somewhere near 2,500 kcals, while for normal adult females with moderate activity they fall around 2,000kcals. But, from my point of view, you should not guide yourself by these values.

Personally, I consume between 1,500 - 1,700 kcals per day and I train heavily many times per week. From the suggestions above, I should be constantly hungry and lose weight (fat and/or muscle) with my strategy. But I am very satisfied with my dietary approach (focusing on ketosis and micronutrient optimization) and my gym performance seems to be constantly improving.

Remember, I often consume less than this amount and I also often have feasting days (which may make up for the apparent caloric deficit).

The major takeaway messages from this lesson:

**1. Find out how much you eat now (in terms of calories).**
**2. Use the same amount of calories as you switch to ketosis.**
**3. You can later adjust (reduce or increase calories) if you want.**

In the next lesson you will learn more about the feeding window of your intermittent fasting strategy.

## Lesson 4 - IF - Feeding Window - Earlier or Late in the Day

If you remember from a past lesson, my IF protocol is 18/6 - most of the days. I fast for 18 hours and eat food in the remaining window of 6 hours. I usually have 2 meals in my feeding window.

My first meal is at 10 A.M. and my second is at 3 P.M. and it lasts for an hour, until 4 P.M. Then I fast for the next 18 hours, from 4 P.M. until 10 A.M. the next day.

From this example, you can conclude that my feeding window is earlier in the day and that I consume no food later in the afternoon or in the evening. From my experiments and for my current approach, this strategy works very well as it allows me to have a resting sleep during the night.

In the past, I experimented with an evening feeding window, but that was mostly when I did not do IF and I was eating 3 times a day.

At that time I was having my last meal at 10 P.M. after my kickboxing practice. It was basically the same big snack I described in a previous lesson.

With that strategy, often times I did not sleep well - waking up multiple times during the night and having recurring nightmares.

However, there are other folks who have done and still do long-term intermittent fasting of 16/8 and have an afternoon/evening feeding window. They do not report having the same problems that I had when I ate at night (but we have to consider that I wasn't doing IF at that time).

Which brings me to the point: I recommend experimenting with both morning and evening feeding windows to see what works best for you.

In the next lesson, you will learn about what's often called to be 'kicked out of ketosis'.

## Lesson 5 - Getting Kicked of Ketosis for Too Much Food During IF's Feeding Window

Getting 'kicked out of ketosis' is an expression you often hear in the community of people who follow a very-low-carbohydrate (ketogenic) diet.

As a refresher, the state of ketosis is when your body mostly uses ketones and fatty acids to create energy.

*Getting kicked out of ketosis* is when your body reverts to using glucose (from carbohydrates) as the main source of energy, the reason being is that you have provided enough substrates for this metabolic state to resume.

When you combine IF and ketosis and when your strategy of feeding includes only two meals (or one - depending on your IF strategy), it means that you have to consume somewhere between 1,500 - 2,500 kcals (or whatever your daily caloric requirements are) in two big meals.

Consuming all your carbohydrates and protein in two meals and consuming so many calories per meal may temporarily kick you out of ketosis due to the short-burst of insulin secretion. This situation could last for a few hours or more.

There is nothing wrong with your strategy if this happens, because you will most likely be out of ketosis for only a few hours and then your body will revert to using mainly ketones and fats for energy for the rest of the hours of your fasting window.

With time and if you are consistent with your strategy and with your feeding and fasting windows, you may be able to tolerate the bigger bouts of calories, carbs, and protein in the same meal and still remain in ketosis all throughout.

In my personal strategy, even after consuming 1,600 kcals in one meal (50-60g of carbs, 40-50g of protein, and the rest of calories coming from fat) I still remain in ketosis.

Another advantage of long-term keto-adaptation is that I don't feel the post-prandial (after meal) energy crash that many people feel. It is probably because I don't secrete too much insulin post meal.

You may also be kicked out of ketosis if you consume alcohol. Once alcohol is in your system, the primary purpose of your body is to metabolize it. It becomes the focus, while macronutrient oxidation is paused. This situation should also be temporary, given that you did not drink sweetened/sugary alcoholic beverages.

Another reason, which somewhat ties to the first point I mentioned, is being kicked out of ketosis for *'falling off the wagon'*, which is an expression that stands for binge eating when on a particular diet. To better understand this, I'll give you an example.

This is the first time you're doing ketosis. You're already 3 weeks in and you've been very strict so far. But you miss your carbohydrate rich foods. You crave for them. One day, things get out of control. You start ravenously consuming sandwiches, pizza, and sweets. You're kicked out of ketosis.

At this moment you should, under no circumstances, blame yourself for anything. It happens to many folks. Remember you're trying to build a lifestyle here, not a limiting temporary diet. So, you should learn from your mistakes.

**What you should do?!**

Try seeking the alternative very-low-carb foods for the carb rich foods you're craving. It's like seeking a fail safe protocol.

Whenever the craving comes (if it comes), you can/could binge eat on the alternative low-carb food and remain in ketosis. This would be a fail safe approach.

Also, it does not matter too much that you've been kicked out of ketosis if you are being consistent with your approach and if this only happens every once in a while (like once a month - or so). This will have a minimal impact on your keto-adaptation status.

The major take-away message is that when you're kicked out of ketosis - for whatever reason being - please learn from your mistakes and get back on the wagon (resume your keto + IF strategy). This is how you build a better and stronger self.

In the next lesson you will learn about some of the exceptions you should allow for with your IF strategy.

Persistent Fat Loss

## Lesson 6 - Social Exceptions for IF

Let's start with a hypothetical situation.

Say that you're following a similar strategy to mine and you're doing **IF + Ketosis**, with an IF feeding window of 6 hours and a fasting window of 18 hours. Your feeding window is in the first part of the day. You only consume food between 10 A.M. and 4 P.M.

Some friends invite you over dinner. It's on them. Your relationship with them is very important to you. You don't want to refuse them and you don't want to go there and be the guy/gal that only drinks water.

The reservation at the restaurant is for 10 P.M. What do you do?

Well, you obviously add an exception to your protocol. You go there, order some keto friendly food and enjoy your time with your friends. You do not have to rigidly stick to your protocol. You might sneak-in one or two glasses of dry red wine (very low carb). But, more about this in a future lesson.

Situations like this one may present themselves from time to time. You have to take them in and make sure they do not impact your long term goals.

For example, if you know you'll gonna have a big dinner at the restaurant, you could skip the 10 A.M. breakfast, and only eat your 3 P.M. meal. This way you're adopting a fail-safe protocol, without even breaking your IF protocol.

With this move, you've temporarily prolonged your fasting window for another 5 hours. Assuming you've not eaten since 4 P.M. the previous day, this means that when you eat today at 3 P.M. you've been fasting for 23 hours.

And this would be a great workaround because you didn't break your protocol, you've improved it. And tomorrow you could simply resume your 10 A.M. to 4 P.M. feeding window.

Hopefully this example gives you an idea about the fact that you should not rigidly stick to your protocol if social situations request your attention and attendance. Friends and family are very important. However, do not make the exception become the rule. Remember, there is a very thin line between the two.

In our next lesson, you will learn about feasting and fasting, a strategy that should maximize your long-term adherence to this combination of protocols, the same way it did to me.

## Lesson 7 - Feasting and Fasting - The Low-Calorie Advantage

Once again, I will start with a personal example.

You already know that I currently consume between 1,500 - 1,700 kcals per day, which is below the daily energy requirements for a person with my physique, by any standards.

However, I would not go so low in calories if I had the slightest feeling of hunger, cravings, or lack of energy. On the contrary, with my strategy, even though it may be hard to believe, I am always satisfied, energetic, and my gym performance is on a constant improvement path.

There are days when I consume even fewer calories because I fast for more than 24 hours. So, after many days in a row on this very low calorie regimen, I tend to start losing weight.

But, I don't want to lose more weight. I've been in maintenance since December 2013. That is why I use the *'fasting and feasting'* protocol.

I fast for 24 hours and then I have a feasting day when I consume 3 or more meals and when my total caloric intake is in the realms of 3,000 - 5,000 kcals. Sometimes, I consume even more calories.

After this feasting day, I return to my regular IF of 18/6. My only major guiding rule for the feasting day is to remain in ketosis. If I am kicked out, that only happens for a couple of hours.

**What can/should you take away from this?**

You should have the hope that combining ketosis with IF will allow you to reach your balance weight in a specific amount of time. And in the mean time you should experience the benefits of ketosis and gradually reduce the caloric intake in a natural way without feeling hungry.

Once you're in maintenance, and possibly even during the weight loss process, you could sneak in some *'fasting and feasting'* days. The effect of these days and the satisfaction you get from them will most likely increase your long-term adherence to this way of life.

In the next lesson I will discuss about alcohol intake, whether it is allowed and if it's allowed, how you can use it to your advantage and not to the detriment of your strategy.

## Lesson 8 - Alcohol Intake - And my Personal Strategy

From what I've seen happening around me and from what I've experienced during my teenage years, there's a very thin line between decent-moderate-therapeutic alcohol intake (if that thing exists) and competitive drinking. You can shift into the wrong direction so easily that you can't even perceive it.

If you enjoy the taste of alcohol, there's a very decent (small) dose that can be therapeutic. Whether it's 1-2 oz. of a spirit drink with lemon juice or sparkling water on the side or 1-2 (not more) glasses of red dry wine once or twice a week (not more often), these may elicit fairly positive effects to your health.

If you cross that line, you get the downsides of alcohol consumption. And it's pretty easy to cross the line when you have friends, family or acquaintances that 'push' you to drink more. But, you should be the one in control!

The small therapeutic dose, if you enjoy the taste of alcohol, can serve as a relaxing tool, one that adds to the atmosphere - when you spend precious time with your closest ones. If you don't enjoy the taste of alcohol, simply avoid consuming it.

### How do I do it?

Whenever you consume alcohol, it becomes the main focus of your metabolism. The process of macronutrient oxidation (breaking down food for energy) is paused. If you have a lot of food in your system at the time of alcohol consumption, that may be shunted into the adipose tissue.

Your body detoxifies/breaks-down alcohol and can use it for energy. But it is mostly empty calories. The biochemistry of this process is boring and uninteresting and I will not describe it in this lesson. So, alcohol should be counted as calories and should add to your daily caloric intake.

I consume 2 glasses of dry red wine once or twice a week. This is not the norm. I went for weeks without consuming alcohol. And I felt fine. In fact, I felt great!

Conversely, I also had multiple days in a row when I consumed 2 glasses of wine per day. I didn't feel as good. I mostly consume red dry wine. Rarely, I drink 2-3 oz. of whisky with 1-2 ice-cubes in it.

For reference, 1 medium size glass (187 ml - or 6.3 fl. oz) of red dry wine (of 12-13% alcohol content) should contain an average of 150-160 kcals. So, two glasses would add 300 - 320 kcals to my daily caloric intake. If I usually consume between 1,500 - 1,700 kcals from food, when I know I will be drinking wine, I slightly reduce my caloric intake with 100-200 kcals for that day.

To avoid nutrients being converted into fat inside my system, I usually consume alcohol after many hours since my last meal. So, if my last meal ends at 4 P.M., I will have my 1-2 glasses of red wine at 10 P.M. (six hours after the last meal). This is kind of a fail safe protocol for alcohol consumption.

Additionally, since there is little food in my system, I need less alcohol intake to feel its effects. Honestly, two glasses are more than enough for me. Consuming three glasses of wine would start make me feel really dizzy. And I would also feel the negative effects next day.

Major take-away messages from this lesson:

**1. If you enjoy alcohol, you can consume it. Use small doses (1-2 servings) of low-carb drinks (dry wine, spirits, vodca, etc).**

**2. To minimize/eliminate the possibility of getting fat, make sure you're in a caloric deficit for that day.**

**3. To minimize/eliminate the possibility of getting fat, try having your servings of alcohol 5-6 hours after you last meal.**

Before moving to Chapter 4, let's have a knowledge check-up!

Persistent Fat Loss

# Chapter 3 - Quiz

## 1. What is the most popular way to enter ketosis?

a) eat many fatty foods and reduce the consumption of carbohydrates
b) eat many carbohydrate rich foods and reduce the consumption of fatty foods
c) eat protein rich foods
d) eat high-carbohydrate foods only

## 2. What are some foods that you should avoid when following a ketogenic diet?

a) processed foods - high in refined carbohydrates and high in fat
b) low-carbohydrate foods
c) high-fat foods
d) low protein foods

## 3. When starting a ketogenic diet, how many calories should you consume?

a) the same that you consumed previous (maintain your daily caloric intake)
b) a few more calories
c) less calories
d) twice the calories

## 4. When doing IF, which feeding window is the best?

a) earlier in the day
b) later in the day
c) there is no consensus
d) mid-day

**5. Should you rigidly strict to your IF strategy even in the face of social situations requiring your attention?**

a) Yes
b) No

**6. What is one strategy that may increase the long-term adherence to the combination of protocols of ketosis and IF?**

a) high-caloric consumption
b) feasting and fasting
c) working out everyday
d) daily low caloric consumption

**7. What happens when you get kicked out of ketosis?**

a) your body resumes to a glucose based metabolism
b) nothing happens
c) you start become very hungry
d) you start burning lean mass for energy

**8. What do you do when you're kicked out of ketosis?**

a) start blaming yourself for committing such a big mistake
b) analyze what happened, learn from your analysis, and try becoming better in the future
c) nothing, just follow a high-carbohydrate diet from then on
d) stop eating food for the next 3 days

**9. What type of alcoholic beverages should you avoid on a ketogenic diet?**

a) cocktails, high-sugar, and sweetened beverages
b) whisky
c) red wine
d) white wine

## 10. What is one ketogenic friendly food?

a) pasta
b) whole wheat bread
c) coconut oil
d) cereals

Persistent Fat Loss

# Chapter 4:
## Workout Basics
## Weights, Aerobic Exercise, Using Equipment or Bodyweight

Welcome to the 4th chapter of this book. So far you've become very familiar with ketosis and intermittent fasting and you've learned about different ways to implement them into your lifestyle. You should be able to design your own meals to promote ketosis and your own convenient IF protocol, whether it's 16/8, 18/6, 20/4 or any different meal timing strategy.

Now, I will provide some insight into the types of exercises that you can do to build muscle and/or simply tone your body. From my experience, I need to tell you that the major requirement to lose fat is to manipulate your diet and meal timing to promote a hormonal background that would achieve these results.

Exercise should not be a weight loss tool. You know this from the countless examples in your own life of friends or acquaintances who hit the gym 5 times a week and do cardio for 1 hour each session, and fail to lose weight.

In Chapter 4 you will find out more about:

1. Home/Gym Exercising
2. Exercising with your Bodyweight, with Weights and/or both
3. The Big 5 Protocol
4. The Big 5 and High Intensity Training
5. The Big 5 for Bodyweight Training
6. The Big 5 for Weights and Machines
7. Want More? How to Adapt The Big 5 Protocol
8. Massive Muscle Build-Up - High Volume - High Intensity Training

9. The Concept of Progressive Loading
10. Traveling and the Resistance Band

Let's start with the very first lesson of the chapter in which you will learn about home and/or gym workouts.

## Lesson 1 - Home or Gym

In a previous lesson I mentioned that there is no exercise requirement for losing fat (from my perspective). The two most important key principles for this purpose are diet and hormonal optimization, which have been widely addressed so far in the book.

Working out should serve as a tool to increase your wellbeing, to tone your muscles, to grow your muscles, and to optimize your brain function. Please understand and take these as my guiding philosophies. Now, back to our main topic.

As you may have guessed, there are many efficient ways to exercise at home or in the gym.

Whatever strategy you may choose is up to your personal preference. Home, in the gym, and/or both. All three are good options.

If you opt in for home workouts, you may do the bodyweight training that is addressed in one of our next lessons.

If you choose to workout at the gym, we will focus on weight lifting and *The Big 5* Protocol.

The frequency of training is another aspect of the workout that is up to you to choose. If you want to train once or twice a week, we'll focus on very high-intensity training, which also happens to be a type of low-volume training.

If your goal is to build muscle and you want to train more than twice a week, we'll focus on high-volume and high-intensity training.

In the next less I will briefly discuss about exercising with your own bodyweight, with weights, and/or using a combination of both of these strategies.

## Lesson 2 - Bodyweight, Weights, or Both

From my personal perspective, there is no actual advantage to either of these two strategies, if you want to build a lean and muscular physique. Of course, if you want to be a competitive body builder you may want to focus on weight training.

If you consider bodyweight training alone, there are many great exercises that you can do at home or in any other place you may find yourself at. You do not require gym equipment. You work with your own bodyweight. This is convenient for people who do not like the gym environment, who may enjoy working outdoors, and also for people who travel a lot.

If you consider working with weights, you may be required to go to the gym. A possible advantage of going to the gym is that you have numerous types of weights, machines, and devices that can work all of the muscle groups of your body. You are also in an environment where you can interact with likeminded people from who you can learn a lot and for whom you yourself can be an inspiring factor.

A combination of the two strategies is possible as well. You can switch between home workouts and gym workouts for your weekly training protocol. You can also work with weights at home (though you'd have to buy them) or you can go to the gym and do bodyweight exercises. It is mostly a matter of preference.

In my personal strategy, I currently do minimal bodyweight training and I focus on going to the gym and lifting weights multiple times per week. I used to do a combination of both strategies, but for now I like to spend my time in the gym.

In the next lesson I will introduce you to *The Big 5 Protocol*, a type of training that I used a lot (and I still use). We will adapt this protocol for bodyweight and for weight workouts.

## Lesson 3 - The Big 5 Protocol

The Big 5, introduced and widely described by Doug McGuff in his book *Body by Science*, is a minimal workout protocol that uses 5 compound movements (that is - targeting big muscle groups and multiple joints - chest, legs, back, biceps, etc). I will become more specific in the upcoming lessons.

This protocol was designed to be extremely efficient as it works the fast twitching muscle fibers (responsible for strength and bulk muscle mass). These are the fibers that grow your muscle.

The other major type of muscle fibers is the slow twitching type, that you work out when you do endurance exercises, such as running or biking.

The major idea behind The Big 5 Protocol is that it has to be done once a week and it should be completed in approximately 12 minutes. Convenient, right?

But, unless done correctly, it does not work to its purpose. Since this protocol involves so little training and so little volume in such a short period of time, the intensity at which the 5 exercises have to be completed is insane.

There is only one set to failure (as many repetitions as you can complete) required for each movement. You have to work with heavy weights and each repetition should be completed as slow as possible. So, it is indeed pretty intense.

I personally started doing The Big 5 Protocol in 2013. It was adapted for gym workouts. It was about the same time I started with ketosis.

In the beginning I trained once a week. It was good enough for getting me in shape. But since ketosis as a metabolic state allows for faster recovery between workouts, I really felt I wanted to be in the gym more than once a week.

And I continued with doing the protocol twice a week. Then I modified it to be similar to a protocol that many bodybuilders use. More details, shortly.

Once again, you have to find/adapt the protocol that fits to your individual needs.

In our next lesson I will discuss about the importance of high intensity training.

## Lesson 4 - The Big 5 and High-Intensity

If you are an athlete who participates in endurance competitions or you just enjoy doing endurance workouts, *ketosis+IF*, if done consistently and for the long-term, will most likely allow you to train more efficiently and for longer, recover faster, and require you to consume nothing but water and some electrolytes during your workouts.

The reason for that is that you will be mostly burning fatty acids and ketones during your workouts.

Keto-adapted elite athletes can burn as much as 1.8g of fat per minute of training compared to 0.8-1g of fat per minute for non-keto-adapted elite athletes (sugar burners). This was well documented in various scientific experiments. Link to Youtube lesson https://www.youtube.com/watch?v=GC1vMBRFiwE

I am not very experienced with endurance training under the combination of these 2 protocols (ketosis and IF).

I did, however, engage in a lot of endurance training for years before becoming ketotic. As of that, in this chapter I will mostly focus on strength training. There are many resources and people that you can follow to learn more about endurance training under ketosis. I will mention some of them in the *Resources* chapter of the book.

The major theme behind The Big 5 protocol is its emphasis on high intensity. Since it has to be done so infrequently and for such a low volume (1 set to failure), the intensity has to be very high to elicit the metabolic and hormonal adaptations that allow you to build muscle and maintain a great physique.

To increase the intensity, this protocol focuses on:

- doing each repetition very slow - (i.e. 20-30 seconds for a repetition)
- using heavy weights - (i.e. - 80%-85% of 1 RM).

**1RM - 1 Rep Max** - is the term used to determine the maximum weight (or load) with which you can complete 1 repetition of any exercise.

For example, my 1 RM for bench press can be 90 kg (~200 pounds). This is the maximum weight (load) with which I can complete 1 repetition on the bench press.

80% of this weight (that is 72kg or ~160 pounds) is what I will use in my Big 5 training.

So, for example, for the bench press I do 1 set of as many repetitions as I can with 72kg (the load). And I will try to do them very slowly. The same principles apply to the rest of the exercises and movements of The Big 5.

If you want to train with your own bodyweight, you will most likely not going to use additional weights, so you will have to focus on doing your repetitions extremely slow. It may be a bit strange and uncomfortable at first, but you will get used to it as you start seeing the results coming.

In the next lesson, I'll give you an example of bodyweight workout for The Big 5.

## Lesson 5 - The Big 5 for Bodyweight

The Big 5, as its name implies, uses 5 movements/exercises per workout. For each of these movements you have to complete 1 set to failure - as many reps as possible, as slow as possible. This is how you exercise your fast twitching muscle fibers to increase your strength and build muscle mass. The workout takes little time to complete, but it is extremely intense.

The 5 movements should include these muscle groups:

- biceps (and triceps)
- chest (and shoulders)
- back
- legs - 2 movements - or 2 sets of the same movement

**1. For biceps** bodyweight workout there's not too much information out there, but here's a very interesting and challenging workout, requiring nothing but your own bodyweight.

It's better if you see it rather than having me trying to explain it in words.

Link https://www.youtube.com/watch?v=kzohU7hbN9I

For triceps, you can do chair dips or bench dips.

Please follow the link to the short explanatory video.

Link https://www.youtube.com/watch?v=tKjcgfu44sI

**2. For chest,** the suggestion is pretty straightforward. Do pushups as slowly as you can.

Additionally, if you want to use weights and make the exercise more intense, you can load a backpack with heavy stuff (or simply with books) and do slow push-ups that way.

You can follow the link for additional chest exercises that you can do at home.

Link https://www.youtube.com/watch?v=P4xXbPhzUrQ

**3. To workout your back** without using weights or equipment, please follow the links. It may not be easy to do these back exercises slowly. But, I challenge you!

Link 2 is a list of short videos that may make things easier (and you can do the back exercises slower and more intense).

Link 1 http://dailyburn.com/life/fitness/no-equipment-back-exercises/

Link 2 http://www.takefitness.net/5-bodyweight-back-exercises-no-equipment-required/

**4. To workout your legs** with your own bodyweight, you can do bodyweight squats. This exercise alone may be enough to fulfill your Big 5 workout needs for this movement.

Additionally, you can follow the link for more bodyweight leg exercises that you can adapt to the Big 5 Protocol.

Link https://www.youtube.com/watch?v=HIdxYCrqLQg

Please remember that for each of these movements you have to do 1 set to failure and try to complete each repetition as slowly as possible. Please do not blindly follow the examples you see in the video links provided. Please adapt them to the protocol - 1 set to failure, very slow movements.

Additionally, you can use the resistance band (search on Amazon for "resistance band" or "resistance tube" and get the 'level 3' or 'intense' version of it). You should find this band at $10. It's very light and convenient to carry around whenever you travel. And you can exercise your entire body with it. But, more on this in a separate lesson.

In the next lesson you will learn about a version of the Big 5 Protocol adapted for gym (weighted) workouts.

Persistent Fat Loss

## Lesson 6 - The Big 5 for Weights and Machines

In this lesson we will adapt the Big 5 Protocol for gym workouts, where you can use both free weights and/or machines when exercising.

To refresh your memory, the movements for this protocol involve the muscles of the:

- biceps (and triceps - indirectly)
- chest (and shoulders - indirectly)
- back
- legs - 2 movements

1. For biceps you can use dumbbells and do dumbbell bicep curls, or you can use the biceps machine.
2. For the chest exercise you can use the barbell bench press, or the chest press machine.
3. For the back exercise you can do the lateral pulldown, do cable rows, or dumbbell rows.
4. For the leg exercise you can do the barbell squat, or use the leg press machine.

Please do a web-search of images of each of these movements. It's much better than having me posting copyrighted pictures here. The same goes with the video links provided in this book. There are many people better than me to explain these movements. I'd rather recommend seeing their videos than recording myself and not doing a job as good as theirs. Back to The Big 5...

Remember, 1 set to failure for each exercise is enough.

When using weights, please remember to use 80% of your 1RM. So, please first determine your 1RM for each movement. If you don't want to do that, you can work with a weight (load) that you can only complete ~5-6 very slow repetitions with.

Here's an example of a full Big 5 workout from *Doug McGuff* himself.

<u>Link</u> https://www.youtube.com/watch?v=5eNBTZiZnLY

Remember, if you're doing it correctly - very slow, 1 set to failure for each exercise, very intense- you only need to do it once a week to see results. A complete workout should last no longer than 12-15 minutes.

In the next lesson, I will show you how you can modify this protocol if you would like to workout more than once a week.

## Lesson 7 - Want More? How to Modify The Big 5

I want to re-emphasize that The Big 5 Protocol is more than enough for most people who only want to tone their bodies, but also for those who want to increase their muscle mass significantly.

But, and here comes the *big but*.

Assume that you enjoy working out a lot, or that you're used to going to the gym multiple times per week, or that you engage in bodybuilding competitions, or that you want to become extremely lean and muscular, or anything in between.

In either of these cases, the Big 5 Protocol can be modified or even replaced with other workout protocols.

Some options you may have:

**1. Do The Big 5 twice a week**. Try maintaining the intensity, the slow repetitions, and the 1 set to failure routine.

**2. Split The Big 5 and train 3-4 times per week.** Use 1 day for 1-2 muscle groups. Add multiple sets (4-5) for each muscle group. Maintain the high intensity (weights and slow repetitions).

**3. Split The Big 5 and train 4-5 times per week.** Use 1 day for 1 muscle group. Do multiple exercises for that muscle group. Maintain a high intensity (heavy weights and slow repetitions).

There are many other possible variations. But you have to always keep in mind to focus on high intensity so that you would recruit your fast twitching muscle fibers in every workout - to build strength and muscle. Otherwise, if you exercise with low weights, many repetitions, fast repetitions, and low intensity you may be recruiting more of your slow twitching muscle fibers (to build endurance) and you may not see the results you expect.

Another point to consider is the time of the day when you will exercise. From a scientific perspective there is no consensus on this matter. I personally find it more convenient to do it early in the morning. You should do it whenever it seems best for you.

Two major recommendations that I have for workout timing:

**1. Do it in a fasted state** (on an empty stomach) - it seems to be more efficient - you can/may have coffee before. For reference, I am almost always at least 16 hours fasted when I workout. If you are not used to this, it may take some time until you can efficiently train in a fasted state.

When you're just starting out with ketosis and IF, this may be more challenging for your body as it is not used to these two strategies combined. Give it time. For me it took more than 6 months of constant ketosis and IF until I recovered the performance I had while being on a higher carbohydrate diet with no IF.

**2. Eat post-workout.** I recommend consuming the bulk of your carbohydrates after your workout as they will be better absorbed by your body and they may have little impact on your ketosis. The same recommendation goes for protein timing.

In the next lesson I will briefly mention one of the most popular strategies that bodybuilders use for their training routines.

## Lesson 8 - Massive-Muscle Build-Up - High Volume and High Intensity

This type of training is somewhat the opposite of The Big 5 Protocol. But, from what I see, to build muscle there is more than one strategy that can work.

Elite bodybuilders usually train 5-7 times per week, and sometimes even twice a day. They use high volume and high intensity in their training.

Bodybuilders use moderate to heavy weights and to increase the intensity of their workouts, they perform many sets of 8-15 repetitions per set. In most workout routines of this kind, they do not do slow repetitions, but often times they do fast repetitions.

The intensity of their workouts is given by the high volume and the high number of reps they do, by the multiple exercises per muscle group, and also by the moderate to heavy weights they use.

Additionally, they spend between 1-3 hours in the gym with each gym session. And this is very different from the 12 minutes - once a week - training that I suggested before.

In the next lesson, I will discuss another important feature of training that you need to have in mind when doing strength training to build muscle.

Persistent Fat Loss

## Lesson 9 - The Concept of Progressive Loading

Whether you're simply doing The Big 5 Protocol once a week or doing a bodybuilder-like type of training where you train multiple times per week, to build bulky muscles and to increase your strength you have to progress your way through weights (the load you use - your working weight).

For The Big 5 Protocol, remember that for each movement, you're doing 1 set to failure for each exercise with a load of ~80% of your 1 RM for that movement. You will mostly be able to do 5-6 slow repetitions until you hit failure.

With time, you will progress. When you are able to do 10 slow repetitions with 80% of your 1 RM, you have to consider increasing the load.

**How do you do it?**

You determine your new 1 RM for the specific movement.

If you use a training protocol that involves more frequent workout sessions per week, and more sets and repetitions ( such as with: bodybuilder-like types of training), you also have to have in mind the principle of progressive loading.

So, when you're able to complete more than 12 repetitions per set with a certain weight and when you feel that the sets you're doing are not intense enough, you have to consider upping the weight (that is, the load) for that exercise.

The new weight should allow you to do no more than 8 repetitions per set. With time, you'll reach the 12 rep mark with the new weight once again. When that happens, you'll have to increase the load once again. I hope you get the point.

This way, as you progress with the load you use, you will most likely become stronger. Becoming stronger almost invariably means having bigger muscles.

With progressive loading, you'll be able to maintain the intensity of your workouts, maintain the 'slow-rep' pace, and also maintain your rep-count in an optimal range for strength and muscle gains (5-6 reps for The Big 5, 8-12 reps for other more frequent protocols).

In our next lesson, we'll move away from massive muscle building and I will introduce you to a tool that I widely use whenever I travel and cannot go to the gym.

## Lesson 10 - Traveling and the Resistance Band

I briefly mentioned this tool in a previous lesson. It is the resistance band. Some people know it as resistance tube. You can find it online under both of these names.

You can get it on Amazon. It costs around $7-$15. It is very convenient to carry around when you travel. It occupies little space and it's very light.

With the resistance band you can do whole body workouts. I enjoy using it mostly when I do biceps and triceps training.

I'd recommend getting the 'high resistance' or 'level 3' version of a resistance tube. It allows for more intense workouts. It may also be better suited for a Big 5 Protocol-like type of training.

If you do not know how to use this tool, please follow the video link for a complete guide to a full body workout with the resistance band.

Link https://www.youtube.com/watch?v=Mx8g7TXJcvQ

Before moving on to Chapter 5, let's do a concept check!

Persistent Fat Loss

# Chapter 4 - Quiz

**1. What is the best place for doing your workouts?**

a) in the gym
b) at home
c) outdoor
d) it is a matter of personal preference

**2. What is the best strategy for exercising?**

a) using only your body weight
b) using weights
c) there is no consensus. It is a matter of personal preference
d) using a combination of weight and bodyweight exercises

**3. What is the workout protocol mostly being discussed in this book?**

a) bodyweight training
b) The Big 5 Protocol
c) outdoor training
d) The 5x5 Protocol

**4. How many times per week you should workout?**

a) as many times as you want. It is up to you to design your preferred workout strategy.
b) once
c) twice
d) six times

**5. How many times per week does the original Big 5 Protocol recommends working out?**

a) twice

b) three times
c) once
d) six times

**6. How many minutes per session was the original Big 5 Protocol initially designed for?**

a) 8 minutes
b) 45 minutes
c) 60 minutes
d) ~12 minutes

**7. What is one of the most used bodybuilding strategy to grow muscle?**

a) The progressive load approach
b) Twice a week workout
c) The Big 5 Protocol once a week
d) Bodyweight training

**8. What is one convenient tool that you can take with you during your travels?**

a) dumbells
b) barbell
c) kickboxing sack
d) the resistance band

**9. Is the Big 5 a very rigid and non-modifiable workout protocol?**

a) Yes
b) No

**10. What is one major feature of the initial Big 5 Protocol?**

Persistent Fat Loss

a) fast repetitions
b) slow-repetitions, high-intensity, and heavy weights
c) low intensity
d) doing cardio every session of the workout

Persistent Fat Loss

# Chapter 5:
## Tools to help you
## Tools I use and their Alternatives

Welcome to the 5th and the last very important chapter of this book. You are already ready to take your health to a superior level through a combination of ketosis and intermittent fasting.

You are also ready to help others do just the same. You have the knowledge, and if you'll be successful in your approach, you will also have the skill.

To help you go along, I will provide some of the tools that I use in my health optimization approach.

One of them is purely for tracking food intake, timing, and everything I put into my mouth.

Another one is to measure ketosis from time to time.

And a third one is to track my exercising routine to know that my progressive loading approach is efficient. These tools are free to use. They also have paid versions that provide you with additional options. Using the free version is enough to achieve optimal results.

In the 5th Chapter of this book you will learn about:

1. Cronometer and Food Tracking
2. Revisiting the Testing Methods for Ketosis
3. JeFit and Workout Tracking
4. Some Supplements to Use

Let's start with the first lesson.

Persistent Fat Loss

## Lesson 1 - Cronometer and Food Tracking

It is called Cronometer and it is a web-based application with a lot of user friendly features for life-logging purposes.

You cannot only use it to track your food, but also to track your exercising routines - though for that purpose I use another tool -, to enter notes, to track water, coffee, and alcohol intake, to track your weight, and many other features.

There is also the smartphone app version of Cronometer, available for iPhone and Android users. I have the Android version, but I mostly use the web version.

Link https://cronometer.com/

Here's how you can use it. I will post a few illustrations and then the explanations for each.

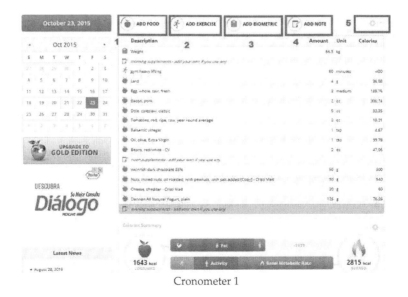

Cronometer 1

# Persistent Fat Loss

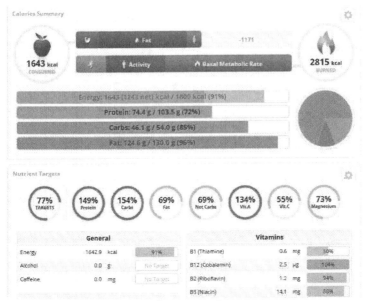

Cronometer 2

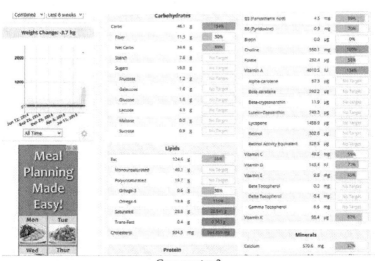

Cronometer 3

**1. In rectangle 1 (illustration 1)** - which I highlighted in red - you have the option to add food. When you click on that, you will be given a list of thousands of foods and products that you can add.

When you click on any particular food item, it will give you a short description of its caloric and macronutrient content. You will be able to add the serving size there.

All simple foods are found in the table. Most packaged foods are also found here. If there is a packaged food you consume and you cannot find it in the list, you can simply add it permanently to the list.

To do this, close the 'add food' menu and go to the upper part of the website where it says 'food'. And use the option 'create new food'. To enter the caloric content and macros for your new food, please look at the labels of that food. But, in most cases, you will not have to do that. The database of this app is very inclusive.

You can see the entries that I made for this example (in illustration 1).

**2. In the red rectangle number 2 (illustration 1)** - you have the option to add your workouts - If there's an activity you cannot find in the list, you can simply use the 'custom' option to add it. To know how many calories your custom exercise will burn in a specific amount of time, you can do a web search.

You can see that for this example I created a custom exercise entry called 'gym' where I burn approximately 400 kcals for my 60 minutes session.

I do not necessarily have to burn all those calories in 60 minutes. Heavy lifting workouts may increase your metabolism for up to 48 hours after completion. So, I may be burning more than 400 kcals as a result of my workout.

**3. In the red rectangle number 3 (illustration 1)** - you have the option to add biometric measurements. You can track your height, weight, blood glucose levels, bodyfat, waist size, total cholesterol, LDL-C, HDL-C, and even ketones! I only use this feature to track my weight. But the availability of options makes it so convenient.

**4. Moving on to the red rectangle number 4 (illustration 1) -** you have the option to add notes to your daily log. I recommend using this feature. It helps you really quantify your life and it's very useful and insightful when you revisit your notes at a future time.

I personally use this feature to track my supplement intake. Supplements can also be added through the 'add food' option - and it may be better to do so because this way you include them to your macronutrient and micronutrient analysis for that specific day. For me, I simply got used to adding them as notes.

**5. The red rectangle number 5 (illustration 1)** - is one of the *settings* buttons. I mostly use it to copy entire days of logs. It's convenient for me to do so because there are many days when I eat the same foods and I have the same entries, so I would not have to add them individually. It saves me time.

I do not track my intake of water, coffee, alcohol and other beverages. I just add a note entry whenever I consume something different than water. For example, when I consume 2 glasses of red wine, I just add a note entry of '2 glasses of red wine at night - 6 hours post meal'. I could also add this through the 'add food' option. But I got used to add it as note.

Right below your entry list (illustration 2) you have a summary of your calories and macros. You can set daily targets (goals) for each of these groups. Below that, you have a more in-depth analysis of the macronutrients, vitamins, and minerals you

127

consumed with your food. Clicking on a specific food entry in your list will give you the in-depth analysis of that food.

The calendar on the right (illustration 3), and also the 'weight change' progression chart right below are two important features to consider. This web/smartphone application has much more attached to it than I can describe here. I only pointed out to you some of its most basic features. And all of them are available with the free version.

There's also a paid version which gives you some more options and features. The major advantage to the paid version is that it give you access to the full history of your entries with which you can do many types of data analysis.

I believe the price for the paid version is approximately $5 per month. Anyway, you will do just fine with the free version only. And I'll let you reserve the privilege of discovering the rest of the features of this app.

Another very similar application (if you don't want to use *Cronometer*) is *MyFitnessPal*.

Link http://www.myfitnesspal.com

In the next lesson, I will review the three most used methods for tracking ketone levels.

Persistent Fat Loss

## Lesson 2 - Revisiting the Testing Methods for Ketosis

As you can remember, you can currently measure the ketone levels in your body in three ways:

**1. Urine Ketones** - With Ketone Strips - $10-$15 for ~50 tests - it takes ~1 minute to test and most of the tests measure Aceto-Acetate.

It is the cheapest way to go. Many advocates of low-carb diets will claim these are the most unreliable tests because as your body gets more efficient to using ketones, it will excrete fewer of them in your urine, so by using the strips you will not know for sure the levels of ketones that are in your blood.

This may be true. But you can use these strips for at least the first couple of weeks of constant ketosis. I am still using them after two years of constant ketosis and they still are very reliable. So, it depends on an individual basis.

To get them, go to Amazon and search for "urine ketone strips".

### 2. Blood Ketones - Blood Ketone Meter

It takes at least $30 to buy the blood ketone monitor and $4-$5 for each test strips. With the blood monitor, you have to prick your finger for a small blood drop, same as you would do with a blood glucose meter. You put the blood on the strip and then you plug the test strip into the ketone monitor and wait for a couple of seconds to get a reading.

The ketone blood monitor system measures BOHB blood levels. It is very accurate, but it is also expensive (device + strips). Once again, for beginners I'd recommend starting with the urine strips.

### 3. Breath Ketones - Breath Ketone Meter

There is at least one good way to measure the ketones in your breath. Remember, when you are in ketosis, you may be excreting acetone (a ketone body). To measure breath ketone levels I know there is a device called *Ketonix*. You can find out more about it on Amazon or by searching for it on the web.

There may be some other tools that are developed for this purpose but I am not familiar with them. For reference, a breath ketone meter may be priced around $100. And it seems to be quite reliable.

I definitely recommend using any of these three methods when starting out with ketosis, because without them - there is no accurate way to know you are actually in this metabolic sate. Measuring ketones helps you determine your limit levels of carbohydrate intake, which is also very important.

In the next lesson, I'll introduce you to *JeFit*, a smartphone application that I use to create and log my workout routines.

## Lesson 3 - JeFit and Workout Tracking

I started using *JeFit*, a web-based and smartphone application, in 2013, a couple of months before starting with ketosis. I did not have a regular exercising routine back then. With time, I became more knowledgeable about workout protocols and I started organizing the way I exercise in a more efficient way.

Tracking your workouts may not be important if your focus is only to tone your muscles. But it may be a necessity if you want to grow your muscle mass.

Without logging your workouts, you may not efficiently do the progressive loading approach I described in a previous lesson. It would be like shooting with blind bullets.

Additionally, if you don't want to use an app for tracking your workouts, you could simply use pen and paper.

As for *JeFit*, there is a free and a paid version of this app. The free version is enough for any of the purposes I mentioned above. Now, let me show you a few of its features.

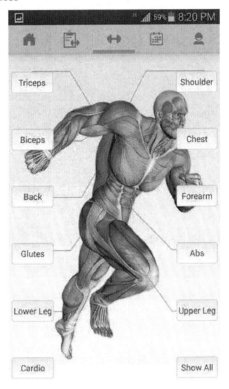

JeFit 1

**1. First of all,** you can and should build a workout routine (that is list of exercises, sets, reps, seconds of pause, etc) for every day of the week you spend in the gym. It will be easier and very convenient to log routines when you're in the gym. This way, you will not be spending too much time on your phone while working out.

Additionally you could use the pen and paper approach when you're in the gym and then plug-in the values of your workout when you get back home. It's up to you to choose.

**As you can see**, it's easy to select exercises for your routine. You can do it by selecting the muscle group and then the

133

specific exercises. If you know the exact name of your exercise (i.e. "wide lateral pulldown") you could simply find it using the search function.

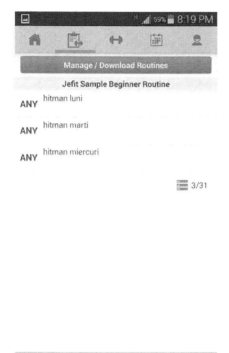

JeFit 2

**2. This is an example of the weekly routines** I have for myself. The first one is for the first workout of the week, the second routine is for the second workout of the week, and the third one is for the third workout of the week.

I usually leave a day of rest between workout days, so in any particular week I would go to the gym on Mondays, Wednesdays, and Fridays. If I go to the gym more frequently during any particular week, I'd simply use routine 1 for the 4th session day in the gym and so on.

I have to emphasize the level of customization that you can apply to all of these routines and even to exercises themselves. This application is extremely complex.

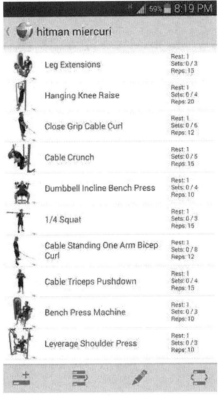

JeFit 3

**3. Here's a sample breakdown** of exercises that I currently have for Routine #3 (workout day #3):

There are 10 exercises. I usually do whole body workouts, where I try to exercises my major muscle groups with every gym session. A different approach is to do split routines and focus on 1-2 muscle groups with each workout.

Here I focus on legs, abs, biceps, chest, triceps, and shoulders. For other routines, I use different exercises where I focus on other muscle groups.

As you can see, there are multiple sets per exercise and no rest (1 sec) between sets. The rep range is 10-15 reps, with more reps for abdominal exercises.

A great feature of the app is that it shows you a short animation of the exercise you are logging. So, it kind of shows you how to do it correctly.

I really enjoy this particular workout routine, which is why I would encourage you to find a specific type of training that you can stick to and build a routine that you can put in your app so that you will be able to log it every time you do it.

Remember, the key point is to focus on progressive loading. Whenever you feel like you can do more reps of an exercise, when you feel you've progressed and the exercise is not as intense, you definitely have to increase the load (weight).

You may guide yourself by the 80% 1 RM principle I discussed in Chapter 4, by the slow-repetition principle, by the 8-12 rep range principle, by the 5-6 rep-range and the 1 set to failure principle, by the high-intensity principle, and so on.

For reference, there are many other similar apps that you can use. You don't have to use *JeFit* if you don't want to. You can search for other apps in the application store of your smartphone or you can use other web-based applications.

In the next lesson, you will learn about a few of the supplements that I'm using and that you may use as well.

Persistent Fat Loss

## Lesson 4 - Some Supplements to Use

I believe that the first layer of focus for optimal fat loss is nutrition optimization: trying to include as many nutrient rich foods to your protocol as possible.

Many ketogenic diets are energy rich, but nutrient poor: because followers focus too much on fat consumption and disregard the inclusion of vitamin, mineral and micronutrient rich foods in their diets (such as plant foods, for example).

As you know from my approach, I try to stay away from that. And I suggest you do the same.

When your nutrition is well optimized, you can think of adding supplements to your protocol. Please consider supplements for what their name implies they are: supplements - that is they should supply a well formulated diet, and not replace it.

They can be extremely contributory to an increased wellbeing. When using supplements, the first focus should be on sourcing. Please make sure they come from a reliable, organic, non-polluted source and please make sure they contain a good amount of the compound/active ingredient you are seeking. Many supplements contain little active ingredients; yet they are filled with additives, preservatives, and toxic chemicals.

Here are some examples of the supplements that I am using:

**1. Magnesium - 600mg/day (organic elemental) - 160% RDA**

My nutrition also contains significant amounts of Mg rich foods.

**2. Prebiotics and Probiotics - 2 pills/day**

They are very beneficial for gut health.

### 3. DHA/EPA - from Cod Liver Oil and Fish Oil

Be very careful when selecting a fish oil supplement. Its source is extremely important. Many supplements come from fish living in polluted waters. You don't want that in your supplement.

Plus, fish oil is easily oxidizable if it's exposed to light and high temperature. You could seek a fish oil supplement that has anti-oxidants in the ingredient list (such as Vitamin E for example).

My DHA/EPA daily intake is approximately: 700 mg EPA/ 500 mg DHA.

A conventional 1,000 mg fish oil gelatin capsule may provide ~18% EPA (180 mg) and 12% DHA (120 mg). You could use 2-3 capsules/day.

### 4. B-Vitamins Complex

### 5. 1 Multivitamin/Multimineral Pill

### 6. Zinc - 50mg/day

### 7. Spirulina and/or Chlorella Powder - 1 tsp

### 8. Alpha Lipoic Acid - 600-900 mg/day.

This one helps with managing blood sugar levels. It is also a very potent anti-oxidant and, possibly, life extending chemical.

There are several other supplements that I use. This is only a short list. For additional information about my strategy, I'd recommend seeing this long post that I did on my Supplements Stack.

<u>Link</u> http://cristivlad.com/supplements-stack-1-what-im-using-and-what-ive-experimented-with/

Next stop, the final chapter! But first, let's do the end of chapter quiz.

Persistent Fat Loss

# Chapter 5 - Quiz

## 1. Do you have to use pen and paper to track your food intake?

a) Yes
b) No

## 2. Do you have to use pen and paper to log your workouts?

a) Yes, this is a must
b) No, but you can do it this way if you want

## 3. What is the tool/software used as example for food tracking in this book?

a) pen and paper
b) MyFitnessPal
c) Cronometer
d) Jefit

## 4. What is the application used in this book for logging workouts?

a) Cronometer
b) MyFitnessPal
c) Jefit
d) Lift

## 5. What is the cheapest way to test ketone levels in the body?

a) urine tests
b) blood ketone meter
c) stool test
d) breath ketone meter

## 6. What is the blood ketone level where ketosis starts?

a) 0.1 mmol/L
b) 0.2 mmol/L
c) 2 mmol/L
d) 0.5 mmol/L

## 7. What is the optimum range for ketone levels in the blood?

a) 0-1 mmol/L
b) 1-1.5 mmol/L
c) 2-5 mmol/L
d) 10-20 mmol/L

## 8. Should supplements replace a well formulated diet?

a) Yes, they may
b) No, they definitely do not have to replace a well formulated diet

## 9. What is characteristic to T1 diabetes patients?

a) high blood sugar levels and high blood ketone levels
b) low blood sugar levels
c) low blood ketone levels
d) low blood sugar levels and low blood ketone levels

## 10. What is a guiding principle when buying supplements?

a) the price
b) making sure they come from a reliable source
c) you should not use supplements
d) ensure that you have at least 1 month of supply

# Chapter 6:
# Further Directions

You have been waiting for this moment for a long time. Now you have everything you need to benefit from the combination of ketosis and intermittent fasting. Moreover, you may be prepared to help others along their journeys as well.

Before giving you further directions and recommendations, I need to repeat something very important:

*I am not a medical doctor and I do not play one on the internet. This book is the result of my personal approach to improving my health. It should be used for information purposes only and if you decide to try implementing some of the concepts from it, I'd recommend discussing this with your physician of confidence.*

In Chapter 6, I will talk about:

1. A Few Books to Start With
2. Some People you could Follow
3. A few Podcasts and Radio Shows you could Subscribe to
4. Leveraging on the Power of Youtube
5. Thank You!

Let's start with the first lesson.

Persistent Fat Loss

## Lesson 1 - A Few Books to Start With

In this lesson I will recommend a few books that can help you deepen your knowledge on ketogenic diets, better nutrition, increased physical performance, as well as on fasting strategies.

### 1. Steve Phinney and Jeff Volek - The Art and Science of Low Carbohydrate Living

This is probably the most insightful book about well formulated ketogenic diets.

### 2. Steve Phinney and Jeff Volek - The Art and Science of Low Carbohydrate Performance

This is the book that will deepen your knowledge on physical performance under long term ketogenic diets. It's very useful in your process of keto-adaptation. I have to say that this book is a must if one of your focuses is to workout with your new lifestyle.

### 3. Terry Wahls - The Wahls Protocol

This is a case study on Multiple Sclerosis reversal with dietary approaches. It is the personal story of the author and it's a very good reference about what a well formulated ketogenic diet should look like.

### 4. Nina Teicholz - The Big Fat Surprise

This is a very insightful book on the science behind ketogenic diets and also on the misguided dietary message that the wide public (us) has followed over the last 5 decades.

## 5. *Doug McGuff - Body by Science*

This is the book from which you will learn all about The Big 5 Protocol and similar routines for efficient muscle building. What I discussed in Chapter 4 is just my application of this protocol. To know the details, you have to read this book.

## 6. *David Perlmutter - Brain Maker*

This is another book that I'd recommend if you want to learn some practical ways to optimize your nutrition for macronutrient and for micronutrient intake and avoid the pitfalls that many folks following ketogenic diets fall into.

Additionally, if you want to become even more familiar with my journey, you can read my book documenting my ketogenic diet experiment, that is *Ketone Power*, and my book on fasting, that is *Periodic Fasting*.

You can find all these resources on Amazon.

I recommend that they should not be the end point of your research, but the starting point. Once you finish with them, follow the *Recommended Readings* lists on the back of these books and also the Recommendations you get from Amazon, if you got the books from that website. Please never stop learning!

In our next lesson, I'll recommend some guiding principles for following other people's advices.

## Lesson 2 - Some People you could Follow

There are many experts out there. And sadly, you know that many of them are *fake*. How do you know that?

**First of all**, you should start asking yourself questions when you see an inconsistency between walking the walk and talking the talk.

This may be easier if you consider following people/experts from the fitness and nutrition industry. You may obviously do not want to follow a fitness expert who is fat, no matter how professional and well sound his talk may be.

**The second** and extremely important suggestion is for you to be aware of the cognitive biases that each of us may fall into.

When we adopt a thought or a guiding principle, we have the tendency to seek only evidence approving those principles and disregard any disconfirming evidence. This is known as the *confirmation bias*.

Please do a web search to learn more about the confirmation bias and other cognitive biases.

And then, please make sure you can spot confirmation biases in the people you may consider following. They may not be a good candidate for your followership if they suffer from these biases.

To have little influence on your decisions, I will not make specific recommendations for people you can follow. I will let you discover them for yourself.

In our next lesson, I will tell you about some of the podcasts and radio shows I listen to in order to further my knowledge on health optimization.

## Lesson 3 - A few Podcasts and Radio Shows you could Subscribe to

I tend to listen to podcasts and radio shows whenever I do unimportant stuff around the house, when I cook, when I clean around, and whenever I have some free time to spare.

The podcasts that I listen to are hosted by folks who, to me, seem that they walk their walk and talk their talk. I enjoy listening to these folks because they also do experiments (they are self-experimenters) and they are good not only at talking.

I also enjoy their shows because they have amazing guests that spark my interest and my attention. Many of them are researchers and doctors.

So, here's the list:

**1. Ben Greenfield** -

Link - http://www.bengreenfieldfitness.com/podcasts/

**2. Dr. Dan Stickler** -

Link - http://ephysiologix.com/podcasts/

**3. Damien Blenkinsopp** -

Link - https://thequantifiedbody.net/author/damien-blenkinsopp/

**4. Dr. Rhonda Patrick** -

Link - http://podcast.foundmyfitness.com/rss.xml

**5. Jesse Lawler -**

<u>Link</u> - http://smartdrugsmarts.com/#

**6. Tim Ferriss -**

<u>Link</u> - http://fourhourworkweek.com/podcast/

You can listen to these shows on the web by following the links provided or you can use a free podcast application on your smartphone and subscribe to these shows. On my Android, I use the app called *Podcast Addicts*.

In our next lesson, you will learn more about the concept of continual/continuous learning.

## Lesson 4 - Leveraging on the Power of Youtube

I am firm believer that learning should never end. It should go beyond the years of formal schooling. And this thought may be more valid today than in any other time in history. Technology and the Internet allow for this.

Today we can learn anything we want at any time. We should feel privileged.

We have this privilege but not many people use it. You see folks spending time on the Internet entertaining themselves with funny videos and with scrolling through social media platforms. There is nothing wrong with that as long as they do not complain about their situation. Each individual can do whatever they want with their time.

This book would have not been made possible were it not for this privilege I am talking about. I would not have had the knowledge, the experience and the results that I achieved with the strategies I combined, had I not devoted my time to massively learning about and applying these concepts.

One of my most powerful tools can be accessed by anyone and everyone. It is called Youtube.

In any particular day, I watch several medical, biochemistry, and nutrition related lessons from Universities from all over the world.

I subscribed to their Youtube channels. I also watch some raw videos of people training in the gym. I try to apply and modify their tactics to fit to my personal needs.

Here are a few channels that I subscribed to:

**University of California Television**
**Khan Academy**
**Albert Einstein College of Medicine**
**Columbia University**
**Crash Course**
**Cornell University**
**Fundamentals of Biochemistry**
**NIHvcast**
**GenomeTV**
**Moof University**
**iBiology**
**Hawthorn University**
**Ted-Ed**
**Talks at Google**
**Bozeman Science**
**The Royal Society**
**The IHMC**

and the list goes on and on.

To find these channels, please go to Youtube and use the search function.

I also follow a few channels of people who do intermittent fasting daily. I am interested to see their experience with this protocol. Two channels are:

**The Hungarian Experiment**
**Kinobody**

They do not do ketosis though, but I like how they designed their lifestyles around IF itself.

Besides watching lessons conferences on Youtube, I also attend courses on the subjects I am mostly interested in on the Coursera website. They are free. They are taught by professors from elite Universities all around the world.

After finishing any Coursera course, you can get a certified diploma for a small fee.

<u>Link</u> http://coursera.org (the link is in the transcript).

There are other sites where you can do online courses. You can find them using your preferred search engine. You just have to search for "online courses for free" or "massive open online courses".

Now, the time has come for me to say goodbye and also to add a few closing remarks.

Persistent Fat Loss

# Thank You!

First of all, thank you for taking the time to reach to the end of this book.

I can now, very confidently, say that you have everything you need to take your health to the next level, to optimize it with the strategies used in this book. You also have lots of tools to help you around and a lot of resources to further build your knowledge and craft your skill. Please use them!

Once you begin to take massive action, implement and adapt these strategies, and once you start seeing the results you've been seeking for so long, you can also start helping others do just the same.

So, my hope is that I've helped you so that you can help yourself and also help other people.

Please, remember these five guiding principles:

**Implement**
**Adapt**
**Improve**
**Never stop learning**
**Enjoy the journey.**

Now, I will not say goodbye. I hate saying goodbye. I will only say:

**I'll see you soon!**

## End of Chapter Quizzes - The Keys

### 1. Chapter 1 Quiz

Key: 1d, 2c, 3a, 4a, 5d, 6c, 7b, 8d, 9b, 10a.

### 2. Chapter 2 Quiz

Key: 1a, 2d, 3a, 4b, 5a, 6c, 7a, 8a, 9c, 10a

### 3. Chapter 3 Quiz

Key: 1a, 2a, 3a, 4c, 5b, 6b, 7a, 8b, 9a, 10c.

### 4. Chapter 4 Quiz

Key: 1d, 2c, 3b, 4a, 5c, 6d, 7a, 8d, 9b, 10b.

### 5. Chapter 5 Quiz

Key: 1b, 2b, 3c, 4c, 5a, 6d, 7c, 8b, 9a, 10b

## About the Author - And Gratitude

Cristian Vlad Zot studies and experiments with nutrition science, neuroscience, exercise physiology, and entrepreneurship (surprisingly).

He holds a Master's Degree in Civil Engineering since 2013, but he did not get a chance to use it yet because at the time of his graduation he was already deep into the rabbit hole...

In his own words:

*I try to gather as much input as possible from my daily activities, analyze it, and come up with solutions that can help me and other people as well. And I thank the divinity for blessing me with the privilege, inspiration, and the time to do what I do.*

Other books from the same author:

*1. Ketone Power - Superfuel for Optimal Mental Health and Ultimate Physical Performance*

*2. T-(Rx) - The Testosterone Protocol - On Achieving True Male Status*

*3. Periodic Fasting - Repair your DNA, Grow Younger, and Learn to Appreciate your Food*

*4. Urban Escape - A Digital Entrepreneur's Travel Guide for New York City*

More at: http://cristivlad.com

Made in the USA
Lexington, KY
31 May 2016